Visual Impairment and Rehabilitation SOURCEBOOK

SECOND EDITION

Disability Series

Visual Impairment and Rehabilitation SOURCEBOOK

SECOND EDITION

Basic Consumer Health Information about Vision Health, Conditions Leading to Visual Impairment, and Treatment and Rehabilitation Options

Along with Information on Benefits and Support Services for Individuals with Visual Impairments and Resources for Additional Help and Information

OMNIGRAPHICS
An imprint of Infobase

Bibliographic Note

Because this page cannot legibly accommodate all the copyright notices, the Bibliographic Note portion of the Preface constitutes an extension of the copyright notice.

* * *

OMNIGRAPHICS
An imprint of Infobase
8 The Green
Suite #19225
Dover, DE 19901
www.infobase.com
James Chambers, *Editorial Director*

* * *

ISBN 978-0-7808-2148-4
E-ISBN 978-0-7808-2149-1

Library of Congress Cataloging-in-Publication Data

Names: Chambers, James, editor.

Title: Visual impairment and rehabilitation sourcebook / edited by James Chambers.

Description: Second edition. | Dover, DE: Omnigraphics, an imprint of Infobase, 2024. | Series: Disability series | Includes index. | Summary: "Provides basic health information about visual impairment, conditions that lead to visual impairment, treatment and rehabilitation for vision impairment, and facts about benefits and support services to people who are visually impaired. Includes an index and resources for additional information"-- Provided by publisher.

Identifiers: LCCN 2024028564 (print) | LCCN 2024028565 (ebook) | ISBN 9780780821484 | ISBN 9780780821491 (eISBN)

Subjects: LCSH: Vision disorders. | People with visual disabilities--Rehabilitation. | People with visual disabilities--Services for.

Classification: LCC RE91.V495 2024 (print) | LCC RE91 (ebook) | DDC 617.7--dc23/eng/20240708

LC record available at https://lccn.loc.gov/2024028564

LC ebook record available at https://lccn.loc.gov/2024028565

This book is printed on acid-free paper meeting the ANSI Z39.48 Standard. The infinity symbol that appears above indicates that the paper in this book meets that standard.

Printed in the United States

Table of Contents

Part 4 | Disability Support for Vision Impairment

Part 5 | Additional Resources

Preface

ABOUT THIS BOOK

Visual impairment encompasses a spectrum of conditions affecting the eyes, optic nerve, or brain, leading to varying degrees of vision loss, ranging from blurred vision or loss of central vision to complete blindness. Age-related eye diseases such as cataracts, glaucoma, and macular degeneration are common causes among adults, while congenital factors can cause vision loss from birth. According to the Centers for Disease Control and Prevention (CDC), approximately 12 million people aged 40 years and older in the United States have vision impairment, including 1 million who are blind. Approximately 6.8 percent of children under 18 in the United States have a diagnosed eye and vision condition, and nearly 3 percent have blindness or vision impairment, defined as having trouble seeing even when wearing glasses or contact lenses.

Visual Impairment and Rehabilitation Sourcebook, Second Edition provides a comprehensive understanding of disability and its effect on daily life in the context of vision loss. It explores specific conditions leading to visual impairment, such as refractive disorders, cataracts, retinal diseases, and congenital disorders. The book addresses public health implications, mental health concerns, and fall prevention among older adults. It offers practical strategies for independent living, including orientation and mobility training, assistive devices, and support systems. Additionally, it discusses managing diabetes to prevent vision loss, surgical interventions, multidisciplinary vision rehabilitation, and technological innovations for low vision and blindness. Key aspects such as mental health, employment rights, and access to education for individuals with visual impairments are addressed. The book concludes with a directory of resources for further assistance and information.

HOW TO USE THIS BOOK

This book is divided into parts and chapters. Parts focus on broad areas of interest; chapters are devoted to single topics within a part.

Part 1: Understanding Disability and Visual Impairment lays the groundwork by defining disability, impairment, and activity limitation. It explores the concept of disability inclusion and identifies common barriers to participation. This part also covers healthy living with visual impairment and managing low vision. Additionally, it discusses the public health implications of vision loss and its effect on mental health, as well as strategies for reducing the risk of falls among older adults.

Part 2: Conditions Leading to Visual Impairment explores specific conditions that contribute to vision loss. It covers refractive disorders such as myopia (nearsightedness), hyperopia (farsightedness), and astigmatism. This part also examines other significant causes, including cataracts, retinal diseases, glaucoma, macular degeneration, and congenital disorders. It provides insights into the causes, effects, and management strategies for these conditions.

Part 3: Treatment and Rehabilitation for Vision Impairment focuses on the assessment, prevention, and treatment of vision loss. It discusses both surgical and nonsurgical interventions, as well as rehabilitation approaches and adaptive living skills. This part covers managing diabetes to prevent vision loss and highlights technological innovations for individuals with low vision and blindness. Additionally, it includes information on Braille services and multidisciplinary rehabilitation strategies to enhance quality of life.

Part 4: Disability Support for Vision Impairment addresses essential aspects of living with vision impairment, such as orientation and mobility training, and disability employment rights. It covers access to special education, government benefits, and various support services for individuals with vision loss. This part also explores transportation options and mobility aids aimed at enhancing independence and mobility for people with visual impairments.

Part 5: Additional Resources includes a directory of organizations providing support for people with visual impairments.

BIBLIOGRAPHIC NOTE

This volume contains documents and excerpts from publications issued by the following U.S. government agencies: ADA.gov; Agency for Healthcare Research and Quality (AHRQ); Centers for Disease Control and Prevention (CDC); Genetic and Rare Diseases Information Center (GARD); MedlinePlus; National Cancer Institute (NCI); National Center on Birth Defects and Developmental Disabilities (NCBDDD); National Eye Institute (NEI); National Institute of Diabetes and Digestive and Kidney Diseases (NIDDK); NIH News in Health; U.S. Department of Education (ED); U.S. Department of Transportation (DOT); U.S. Equal Employment Opportunity Commission (EEOC); and U.S. Social Security Administration (SSA).

It also contains original material produced by Infobase.

ABOUT THE *DISABILITY SERIES*

At the request of librarians serving the one in four Americans living with a disability, as well as those seeking information to comprehend, navigate, and manage such conditions, the *Disability Series* was developed as a specialized collection within Omnigraphics' *Health Reference Series*. Each volume comprehensively addresses a specific topic chosen based on the needs and interests of these patrons. These volumes offer authoritative health information, serving as a reliable resource for librarians to equip consumers with the necessary facts to take charge of their well-being. This empowers individuals to better understand and address health challenges faced by themselves, family members, or loved ones. Patrons in search of this information can find answers in the *Disability Series*. The *Series*, however, is not designed for diagnosing disabilities, prescribing treatments, or substituting the health-care provider-patient relationship. Anyone concerned about medical symptoms, the potential for disability, or illness is encouraged to seek professional care from an appropriate health-care provider.

If you have suggestions for future *Disability Series* topics, please email us at: custserv@infobaselearning.com.

A NOTE ABOUT SPELLING AND STYLE

Disability Series editors use *Stedman's Medical Dictionary* as an authority for questions related to the spelling of medical terms and *The Chicago Manual of Style* for questions related to grammatical structures, punctuation, and other editorial concerns. Consistent adherence is not always possible, however, because the individual volumes within the *Series* include many documents from a wide variety of different producers, and the editor's primary goal is to present material from each source as accurately as is possible. This sometimes means that information in different chapters or sections may follow other guidelines and alternate spelling authorities. For example, occasionally a copyright holder may require that eponymous terms be shown in possessive forms (Crohn's disease vs. Crohn disease) or that British spelling norms be retained (leukaemia vs. leukemia).

Part 1 | Understanding Disability and Visual Impairment

Chapter 1 | **Impairment, Activity Limitation, and Participation Restriction**

Chapter Contents

Section 1.1 | What Are Disability, Impairment, and Activity Limitation?

WHAT IS DISABILITY?

A disability is any condition of the body or mind (impairment) that makes it more difficult for a person with the condition to do certain activities (activity limitation) and interact with the world around them (participation restrictions).

There are many types of disabilities, such as those that affect a person's:

- vision
- movement
- thinking
- remembering
- learning
- communicating
- hearing
- mental health
- social relationships

Although "people with disabilities" sometimes refers to a single population, it actually encompasses a diverse group of people with a wide range of needs. Two people with the same type of disability can be affected in very different ways. Some disabilities may be hidden or not easy to see.

DIMENSIONS OF DISABILITY

According to the World Health Organization (WHO), disability has three dimensions:

1. Impairment in a person's body structure or function, or mental functioning. Examples of impairments include loss of a limb, loss of vision, or memory loss.
2. Activity limitation, such as difficulty seeing, hearing, walking, or problem-solving.
3. Participation restrictions in normal daily activities, such as working, engaging in social and recreational activities, and obtaining health care and preventive services.

CAUSES OF DISABILITY

Disability can be:

- related to conditions present at birth and may affect functions later in life, including cognition (memory, learning, and understanding), mobility (moving around in the environment), vision, hearing, behavior, and other areas. These conditions may be:
  - disorders in single genes (e.g., Duchenne muscular dystrophy (DMD))
  - disorders of chromosomes (e.g., Down syndrome)
  - the result of the mother's exposure during pregnancy to infections (e.g., rubella) or substances, such as alcohol or cigarettes
- associated with developmental conditions that become apparent during childhood (e.g., autism spectrum disorder and attention deficit hyperactivity disorder (ADHD))
- related to an injury (e.g., traumatic brain injury or spinal cord injury)
- associated with a long-standing condition (e.g., diabetes), which can cause a disability such as vision loss, nerve damage, or limb loss
- progressive (e.g., muscular dystrophy), static (e.g., limb loss), or intermittent (e.g., some forms of multiple sclerosis (MS))

WHAT IS IMPAIRMENT?

Impairment is an absence of or significant difference in a person's body structure or function, or mental functioning. For example, problems in the structure of the brain can result in difficulty with mental functions, or problems with the structure of the eyes or ears can result in difficulty with the functions of vision or hearing.

- **Structural impairments are significant problems with an internal or external component of the body**. Examples include a type of nerve damage that can result in MS, or a complete loss of a body component, as when a limb has been amputated.

- **Functional impairments include the complete or partial loss of function of a body part.** Examples include pain that does not go away or joints that no longer move easily.

DIFFERENCE BETWEEN ACTIVITY LIMITATION AND PARTICIPATION RESTRICTION

The World Health Organization (WHO) published the International Classification of Functioning (ICF), Disability, and Health in 2001. The ICF provides a standard language for classifying body function and structure, activity, participation levels, and conditions in the world around that influence health. This description helps to assess the health, functioning, activities, and factors in the environment that either help or create barriers for people to fully participate in society.

According to the ICF:

- Activity is the execution of a task or action by an individual.
- Participation is a person's involvement in a life situation.

The ICF acknowledges that the distinction between these two categories is somewhat unclear and combines them, although, generally, activities occur at a personal level and participation involves engagement in life roles, such as employment, education, or relationships. Activity limitations and participation restrictions refer to difficulties an individual experiences in performing tasks and engaging in social roles. Activities and participation can be made easier or more difficult due to environmental factors, such as technology, support and relationships, services, policies, or the beliefs of others.

The ICF includes the following in the categories of activities and participation:

- learning and applying knowledge
- managing tasks and demands
- mobility (moving and maintaining body positions, handling and moving objects, moving around in the environment, moving around using transportation)
- managing self-care tasks
- managing domestic life

- establishing and managing interpersonal relationships and interactions
- engaging in major life areas (education, employment, managing money or finances)
- engaging in community, social, and civic life

It is crucial to improve conditions in communities by providing accommodations that decrease or eliminate activity limitations and participation restrictions for people with disabilities, allowing them to participate in the roles and activities of everyday life.[1]

Section 1.2 | Disability Inclusion

WHAT IS DISABILITY INCLUSION?

Disability inclusion refers to including people with disabilities in everyday activities and encouraging them to have roles similar to their peers who do not have a disability. This involves more than simply encouraging people; it requires ensuring that adequate policies and practices are in effect in a community or organization.

Inclusion should lead to increased participation in socially expected life roles and activities—such as being a student, worker, friend, community member, patient, spouse, partner, or parent.

Socially expected activities may also include engaging in social activities, using public resources such as transportation and libraries, moving about within communities, receiving adequate health care, having relationships, and enjoying other day-to-day activities.

DISABILITY INCLUSION AND THE HEALTH OF PEOPLE WITH DISABILITIES

Disability inclusion allows people with disabilities to take advantage of the benefits of the same health promotion and prevention

[1] National Center on Birth Defects and Developmental Disabilities (NCBDDD), "Disability and Health Overview," Centers for Disease Control and Prevention (CDC), April 3, 2024. Available online. URL: www.cdc.gov/ncbddd/disabilityandhealth/disability.html. Accessed August 2, 2024.

activities experienced by people without disabilities. Examples of these activities include:

- education and counseling programs that promote physical activity, improve nutrition, or reduce the use of tobacco, alcohol, or drugs
- blood pressure and cholesterol assessments during annual health exams and screenings for illnesses such as cancer, diabetes, and heart disease

Including people with disabilities in these activities begins with identifying and eliminating barriers to their participation.

WHY IS THIS IMPORTANT?

Disability affects approximately 61 million, or nearly one in four (26%), people in the United States living in communities. Disability affects more than 1 billion people worldwide. According to the United Nations Convention on the Rights of Persons with Disabilities, people:

> *. . . with disabilities include those who have long-term physical, mental, intellectual or sensory [such as hearing or vision] impairments which in interaction with various barriers may hinder their full and effective participation in society on an equal basis with others.*

People with disabilities experience significant disadvantages regarding health, such as:

- Adults with disabilities are three times more likely to have heart disease, stroke, diabetes, or cancer than adults without disabilities.
- Adults with disabilities are more likely than adults without disabilities to be current smokers.
- Women with disabilities are less likely than women without disabilities to have received a breast cancer x-ray test (mammogram) during the past two years.

Although disability is often associated with health conditions (such as arthritis, mental, or emotional conditions) or events (such as injuries), the functioning, health, independence, and engagement in society of people with disabilities can vary significantly depending on several factors:

- severity of the underlying impairment
- social, political, and cultural influences and expectations
- aspects of natural and built surroundings
- availability of assistive technology and devices
- family and community support and engagement

Disability inclusion means understanding the relationship between how people function and how they participate in society and ensuring that everybody has the same opportunities to participate in every aspect of life to the best of their abilities and desires. By recognizing and eliminating barriers, we can improve the health, independence, and social engagement of people with disabilities, enabling them to lead fulfilling lives.[1]

Section 1.3 | Common Barriers to Participation

Nearly everyone faces hardships and difficulties at one time or another. However, for people with disabilities, barriers can be more frequent and have a greater effect. The World Health Organization (WHO) describes barriers as more than just physical obstacles. According to the WHO, barriers are:

Factors in a person's environment that, through their absence or presence, limit functioning and create disability. These include aspects such as:

- a physical environment that is not accessible
- lack of relevant assistive technology (assistive, adaptive, and rehabilitative devices)
- negative attitudes of people toward disability
- services, systems, and policies that are either nonexistent or that hinder the involvement of all people with a health condition in all areas of life.

[1] National Center on Birth Defects and Developmental Disabilities (NCBDDD), "Disability Inclusion," Centers for Disease Control and Prevention (CDC), September 16, 2020. Available online. URL: www.cdc.gov/ncbddd/disabilityandhealth/disability-inclusion.html. Accessed August 2, 2024.

Often, multiple barriers can make it extremely difficult or even impossible for people with disabilities to function. Here are the seven most common barriers, which often occur simultaneously:

- attitudinal
- communication
- physical
- policy
- programmatic
- social
- transportation

ATTITUDINAL BARRIERS

Attitudinal barriers are the most basic and contribute to other barriers. For example, some people may not be aware that difficulties in getting to or entering a place can limit a person with a disability from participating in everyday life and common daily activities. Examples of attitudinal barriers include:

- **Stereotyping**. People sometimes stereotype those with disabilities, assuming their quality of life (QOL) is poor or that they are unhealthy because of their impairments.
- **Stigma, prejudice, and discrimination**. These attitudes may stem from societal ideas related to disability, such as viewing it as a personal tragedy, something needing a cure or prevention, a punishment for wrongdoing, or an indication of a lack of ability to behave as expected in society.

Today, society's understanding of disability is improving as we recognize "disability" as what occurs when a person's functional needs are not addressed in their physical and social environment. By not considering disability a personal deficit or shortcoming and instead thinking of it as a social responsibility, all people, including those with disabilities, can be supported to live independent and full lives. This makes it easier to recognize and address challenges that all people experience.

COMMUNICATION BARRIERS

Communication barriers are experienced by people who have disabilities affecting hearing, speaking, reading, writing, or understanding and who use different ways to communicate than those without these disabilities. Examples of communication barriers include:

- Written health promotion messages with barriers that prevent people with vision impairments from receiving the message. These include:
  - use of small print or lack of large-print versions of material
  - no Braille or versions for people who use screen readers
- Auditory health messages may be inaccessible to people with hearing impairments, including:
  - videos without captioning
  - oral communications without accompanying manual interpretation (such as American Sign Language (ASL))
- The use of technical language, long sentences, and words with many syllables may significantly hinder understanding for people with cognitive impairments.

PHYSICAL BARRIERS

Physical barriers are structural obstacles in natural or manmade environments that prevent or block mobility (moving around in the environment) or access. Examples of physical barriers include:

- steps and curbs that block a person with mobility impairment from entering a building or using a sidewalk
- mammography equipment that requires a woman with a mobility impairment to stand
- absence of a weight scale that accommodates wheelchairs or others who have difficulty stepping up

POLICY BARRIERS

Policy barriers are frequently related to a lack of awareness or enforcement of existing laws and regulations that require programs and activities to be accessible to people with disabilities. Examples of policy barriers include:

- denying qualified individuals with disabilities the opportunity to participate in or benefit from federally funded programs, services, or other benefits
- denying individuals with disabilities access to programs, services, benefits, or opportunities to participate due to physical barriers
- denying reasonable accommodations to qualified individuals with disabilities, preventing them from performing the essential functions of the job for which they have applied or have been hired

PROGRAMMATIC BARRIERS

Programmatic barriers limit the effective delivery of a public health or health-care program for people with different types of impairments. Examples of programmatic barriers include:

- inconvenient scheduling
- lack of accessible equipment (such as mammography screening equipment)
- insufficient time set aside for medical examinations and procedures
- little or no communication with patients or participants
- providers' attitudes, knowledge, and understanding of people with disabilities

SOCIAL BARRIERS

Social barriers are related to the conditions in which people are born, grow, live, learn, work, and age—also known as "social determinants of health"—which can contribute to decreased functioning among people with disabilities. Examples of social barriers include:

- People with disabilities are far less likely to be employed. In 2017, 35.5 percent of people with disabilities, aged 18–64 years, were employed, compared to 76.5 percent of people without disabilities.

- Adults aged 18 years and older with disabilities are less likely to have completed high school compared to their peers without disabilities (22.3% compared to 10.1%).
- People with disabilities are more likely to have an income of less than $15,000 compared to people without disabilities (22.3% compared to 7.3%).
- Children with disabilities are almost four times more likely to experience violence than children without disabilities.

TRANSPORTATION BARRIERS

Transportation barriers are due to a lack of adequate transportation that interferes with a person's ability to be independent and function in society. Examples of transportation barriers include:

- lack of access to accessible or convenient transportation for people who are not able to drive due to vision or cognitive impairments
- public transportation that may be unavailable or located at inconvenient distances or locations

Understanding and addressing these barriers is crucial for promoting inclusivity and ensuring that all individuals, regardless of their abilities, have equal opportunities to participate in society.[1]

[1] National Center on Birth Defects and Developmental Disabilities (NCBDDD), "Common Barriers to Participation Experienced by People with Disabilities," Centers for Disease Control and Prevention (CDC), May 2, 2024. Available online. URL: www.cdc.gov/ncbddd/disabilityandhealth/disability-barriers.html. Accessed August 2, 2024.

Chapter 2 | **Healthy Living with Visual Impairment**

People with disabilities, including those with visual impairments, need health care and health programs for the same reasons as everyone else—to stay well, active, and part of the community.

Having a disability does not mean a person is not healthy or cannot be healthy. Being healthy means the same for all of us—getting and staying well to lead full, active lives. This means having the tools and information to make healthy choices and knowing how to prevent illness.

For people with disabilities, it also means knowing that health problems related to their condition can be treated. These problems, also called "secondary conditions," can include pain, depression, and a greater risk of certain illnesses.

To be healthy, people with disabilities require health care that meets their needs as a whole person, not just as a person with a disability. Most people, with or without disabilities, can stay healthy by learning about and living healthy lifestyles.

LEADING A LONG AND HEALTHY LIFE

Although people with disabilities sometimes have a harder time getting and staying healthy than those without disabilities, there are things we can all do to get and stay healthy.

Following are few tips for leading a long and healthy life:

- **Be physically active every day**. Engage in activities that keep you moving and active.
- **Eat healthy foods in healthy portions**. Choose nutritious foods and maintain balanced meals.
- **Do not get too much sun**. Protect your skin by using sunscreen and wearing protective clothing.

- **Do not smoke**. Avoid tobacco products to reduce health risks.
- **Use medicines wisely**. Follow prescriptions and medical advice carefully.
- **If you drink alcoholic beverages, drink in moderation**. Limit alcohol intake to reduce health risks.
- **Get help for substance abuse**. Seek support for any substance abuse issues.
- **Stay in touch with family and friends**. Maintain strong social connections.
- **If you need help, talk with your health-care professional**. Seek medical advice and support when necessary.

GETTING THE BEST POSSIBLE HEALTH CARE

People with disabilities, including those with visual impairments, must get the care and services they need to help them be healthy.

If you have a disability, there are many things you can do to ensure you are getting the best possible health care:

- **Know your body**. Be aware of how you feel when you are well and when you are not.
- **Communicate your concerns**. Talk openly with your health-care professional about your concerns.
- **Find health-care professionals you are comfortable with in your area**. You are more likely to visit the doctor and obtain health care this way.
- **Check for accessibility**. Ensure you can physically access your health-care professional's office, including ramps or elevators if needed.
- **Check for necessary equipment**. Ensure your health-care professional's office has accessible equipment, such as an accessible scale or examining table.
- **Ask for help from office staff if needed**. Workers at your doctor's office can help you coordinate your visits.
- **Prepare for visits**. Think about your questions and health concerns before you visit your health-care professional.
- **Bring your health records with you**. It ensures that your health-care providers have all the necessary information to offer you the best possible care.

- **Take a friend with you if you are concerned you might not remember all your questions or what the health-care professional says.**
- **Get it in writing.** Write down or have someone write down what the health-care professional says. Request information in accessible formats if needed.

PHYSICAL ACTIVITY

Adults of all shapes, sizes, and abilities, including those with visual impairments, can benefit from being physically active. For important health benefits, all adults should do both aerobic and muscle-strengthening physical activities. Regular aerobic physical activity increases heart and lung functions; improves daily living activities and independence; decreases the chances of developing chronic diseases; and improves mental health.

Adults with disabilities should try to get at least 2 hours and 30 minutes (150 minutes) a week of moderate-intensity aerobic physical activity (i.e., brisk walking; wheeling oneself in a wheelchair) or at least 1 hour and 15 minutes (75 minutes) a week of vigorous-intensity aerobic physical activity (i.e., jogging, wheelchair basketball) or a mix of both moderate- and vigorous-intensity aerobic physical activities each week. A rule of thumb is that one minute of vigorous-intensity activity is about the same as two minutes of moderate-intensity activity. They should avoid inactivity as some physical activity is better than none.

Muscle-strengthening activities should be moderate and high intensity and involve all major muscle groups on two or more days a week (e.g., working with resistance bands or adapted yoga), as these activities provide additional health benefits. All children and adolescents should do one hour (60 minutes) or more of physical activity each day.

If a person with a disability cannot meet the physical activity guidelines, they should engage in regular physical activity based on their abilities and should avoid inactivity. Adults with disabilities should talk to their health-care provider about the amounts and types of physical activity that are appropriate for their abilities.

Tips for Getting Fit

- Talk to your doctor about how much and what kind of physical activity is right for you.
- Find opportunities to increase physical activity regularly to meet your needs and abilities.
- Start slowly, based on your abilities and fitness level (e.g., be active for at least 10 minutes at a time, and slowly increase activity over several weeks, if necessary).
- Avoid inactivity—some activity is better than none!

ABUSE AND VIOLENCE OF PEOPLE WITH DISABILITIES

People with disabilities are at greater risk of abuse, violence, and harm than those without disabilities. This is called "victimization." Victimization is harm caused on purpose. It is not an "accident" and can happen anywhere. The two most common places where victimization occurs are in hospitals and homes.

Victimization includes:

- physical violence with or without a weapon
- sexual violence of any kind, including rape
- emotional abuse, including verbal attacks or being humiliated
- neglect of personal needs for daily life, including medical care or equipment

In the United States, people with disabilities are 4–10 times more likely to be victimized than those without disabilities. Children with disabilities are more than twice as likely to be victimized as children without disabilities. Researchers found that 11.5 percent of adults with a disability were victims of sexual assault versus 3.9 percent of adults without disabilities. In addition, 13.0 percent of people with disabilities were victims of attempted sexual assault compared to 5.7 percent without disabilities.

Victims usually know the person who harms them. They can be health-care workers, intimate partners, or family members. More men than women cause harm to people with disabilities. If you or someone you love is being victimized, help is available.

- Dial 911 if you need immediate assistance.
- Call the National Domestic Violence Hotline (www.thehotline.org) at 800-799-SAFE (7233) or text "START" to 88788.

SEXUAL HEALTH AND SEXUALITY

Health-care professionals and people with disabilities should feel comfortable talking to each other about sexual health and sexuality. People with disabilities can ask their doctor questions about sexuality, sexual functioning, contraceptives, and reproductive concerns.

MENTAL HEALTH AND WELL-BEING

For everyone, overall mental health and well-being are essential. Mental health is how we think, feel, and act as we cope with life. People need to feel good about their lives and value themselves.

All people, including those with visual impairments, might feel isolated from others or have low self-esteem. They may be depressed. There are different ways to treat depression. Exercise may be effective for some people. Counseling, medication, or both might also be needed.

Everyone feels worried, anxious, sad, or stressed sometimes. If these feelings do not go away, and they interfere with your daily life, you should talk with other people about your feelings, such as a family member or health-care professional.[1]

[1] National Center on Birth Defects and Developmental Disabilities (NCBDDD), "Disability and Health Healthy Living," Centers for Disease Control and Prevention (CDC), May 2, 2024. Available online. URL: www.cdc.gov/ncbddd/disabilityandhealth/healthyliving.html. Accessed August 2, 2024.

Chapter 3 | **Understanding and Managing Low Vision**

WHAT IS LOW VISION?

Low vision is a vision problem that makes it hard to do everyday activities. It cannot be fixed with glasses, contact lenses, or other standard treatments such as medicine or surgery.

You may have low vision if you cannot see well enough to do things such as:

- **Read.** Difficulty reading books, newspapers, or digital screens.
- **Drive.** Inability to drive safely or legally.
- **Recognize people's faces.** Challenges in identifying familiar faces.
- **Tell colors apart.** Difficulty distinguishing between colors.
- **See your television or computer screen clearly.** Blurred or unclear view of screens.

WHAT ARE THE TYPES OF LOW VISION?

The type of low vision you have depends on the disease or condition that caused it. The most common types of low vision include:

- **Central vision loss.** Inability to see things in the center of your vision.
- **Peripheral vision loss.** Difficulty seeing things out of the corners of your eyes.
- **Night blindness.** Difficulty seeing in low light or darkness.
- **Blurry or hazy vision.** A general lack of clarity in vision.

WHAT CAUSES LOW VISION?

Many eye conditions can cause low vision. The most common causes include:

- **Age-related macular degeneration (AMD).** A condition that affects the central part of the retina.
- **Cataracts.** Clouding of the eye's lens.
- **Diabetic retinopathy (DR).** Vision loss caused by diabetes.
- **Glaucoma.** A group of eye conditions that damage the optic nerve.

Low vision is more common in older adults because many of the diseases that can cause it are more prevalent in this age group. However, aging does not cause low vision on its own. Eye and brain injuries, as well as certain genetic disorders, can also cause low vision.

HOW WILL YOUR DOCTOR CHECK FOR LOW VISION?

Your doctor can check for low vision as part of a dilated eye exam, which is simple and painless. During the exam, your doctor will ask you to read letters that are up close and far away and check whether you can see things in the center and at the edges of your vision.

They will give you eye drops to dilate (widen) your pupils and check for other eye problems, including conditions that could cause low vision.

WHAT IS THE TREATMENT FOR LOW VISION?

Unfortunately, low vision is usually permanent. Eyeglasses, medicine, and surgery typically cannot cure low vision, but sometimes they can improve vision, help you perform everyday activities more easily, or prevent further vision loss.

Treatment options will depend on the specific eye condition that caused your low vision. Consult your doctor to learn about any treatments that could improve your vision or help protect your remaining vision.

HOW CAN YOU MAKE THE MOST OF YOUR REMAINING SIGHT?

If you have low vision, there are ways to make the most of your vision and continue enjoying activities you love.

For Minor Vision Loss

- Use brighter lights at home or work to improve visibility.
- Wear anti-glare sunglasses to reduce discomfort from bright light.
- Use a magnifying lens for reading and other close-up activities.

For Significant Vision Loss

If your vision loss interferes with daily activities, consider vision rehabilitation. A specialist can help you adapt to your vision loss, offering:

- training on how to use a magnifying device for reading
- guidance for setting up your home to facilitate movement and safety
- resources to help you cope with vision loss[1]

[1] "At a Glance: Low Vision," National Eye Institute (NEI), November 15, 2023. Available online. URL: www.nei.nih.gov/learn-about-eye-health/eye-conditions-and-diseases/low-vision. Accessed August 3, 2024.

Chapter 4 | **Color Blindness (Color Vision Deficiency)**

WHAT IS COLOR BLINDNESS?

Color blindness, or color vision deficiency, means seeing colors differently than most people. It usually makes it hard to distinguish between certain colors. While there is no cure, special glasses and contact lenses can help people differentiate colors. Most individuals with color vision deficiency do not experience significant problems in their daily lives.

WHAT ARE THE TYPES OF COLOR VISION DEFICIENCY?

- **Red-green color blindness.** The most common type, making it difficult to tell the difference between red and green.
- **Blue-yellow color blindness.** Another type, causing blue and yellow to appear similar.
- **Complete color blindness.** A rare condition where no color is seen at all.

WHAT ARE THE SYMPTOMS OF COLOR VISION DEFICIENCY?

The main symptom is difficulty in seeing colors as most people do. This may manifest as:

- trouble distinguishing between different colors
- difficulty perceiving the brightness of colors
- challenges in identifying different shades of colors

Symptoms can be so mild that they often go unnoticed, and many people adjust to their unique color perception. Severe cases might also involve other symptoms, such as quick side-to-side eye movements (nystagmus) or sensitivity to light.

ARE YOU AT RISK FOR COLOR VISION DEFICIENCY?

Certain factors increase the risk of color vision deficiency, including:

- being male (higher risk compared to females)
- family history of color vision deficiency
- certain eye diseases
- health conditions such as diabetes, Alzheimer disease (AD), or multiple sclerosis (MS)
- use of certain medications
- being white

If you suspect color vision deficiency, consult your eye doctor for an evaluation.

WHAT CAUSES COLOR VISION DEFICIENCY?

Most cases of color vision deficiency are genetic and present from birth. However, it can also result from:

- **Retinal injuries.** Such as retinal detachment.
- **Eye injuries.** Particularly those caused by lasers.
- **Brain injuries.** Including specific tumors affecting the optic nerve or brain.
- **Aging.** Often linked to conditions such as cataracts.

HOW CAN YOU FIND OUT IF YOU HAVE COLOR DEFICIENCY?

Eye doctors can diagnose color vision deficiency with a simple test. One common method involves showing a circle of colored dots with a hidden shape or number. People without color vision deficiency can easily see the shape, while those with the condition struggle to identify it.

WHAT IS THE TREATMENT FOR COLOR VISION DEFICIENCY?

There is no cure for inherited color vision deficiency, but most people adapt to it. Children and adults may need support in certain activities, such as schoolwork or jobs that require color differentiation.

If the deficiency is due to another health issue, treating the underlying condition can help. For medication-induced cases, dosage adjustments or alternative treatments may be recommended.

Options to assist with color vision deficiency include:

- **Glasses and contacts**. Special lenses can help differentiate colors by enhancing contrast.
- **Visual aids**. Apps that identify colors in photos can be useful.

WHAT IS THE LATEST RESEARCH ON COLOR VISION DEFICIENCY?

Recent research suggests gene therapies may offer promising treatments for severe types of color vision deficiency by altering genes in specific locations.[1]

[1] "At a Glance: Color Blindness," National Eye Institute (NEI), November 15, 2023. Available online. URL: www.nei.nih.gov/learn-about-eye-health/eye-conditions-and-diseases/color-blindness. Accessed August 3, 2024.

Chapter 5 | **Understanding and Addressing Vision Loss**

FAST FACTS: VISION LOSS

Vision Loss in the United States

Vision loss ranks among the top 10 causes of disability in the United States. Approximately, 7 million Americans have vision impairment, including 1 million who are blind. These numbers are expected to double by 2050 due to population aging and increases in chronic diseases that can lead to vision loss.

Vision Loss and Age

Approximately, 12 million people aged 40 years and older in the United States have vision impairment, including 1 million with blindness. As of 2012, 4.2 million Americans aged 40 or older have uncorrectable vision impairment. This number is predicted to more than double by 2050 due to the rapidly aging population and the rise in chronic conditions, such as diabetes, which can lead to vision loss. Approximately, 6.8 percent of children under 18 in the United States have a diagnosed eye and vision condition. Nearly 3 percent of children under 18 years have blindness or vision impairment, defined as having trouble seeing even when wearing glasses or contact lenses.

Vision Disabilities

Vision disability is one of the top 10 disabilities among adults 18 years and older and is one of the most prevalent disabling conditions among children. Early detection and timely treatment of eye conditions, such as DR, can be highly effective. Ninety percent of blindness caused by diabetes in U.S. adults is preventable. Vision loss results in substantial social and economic costs, including significant disability, loss of productivity, and decreased quality of life (QOL).

Nationwide Effects of Vision Loss

An estimated 93 million adults in the United States are at high risk for serious vision loss, but only half visited an eye doctor in the past 12 months. Early detection and treatment can often prevent or delay vision loss. The economic cost of major vision problems is estimated to be $373 billion by 2050. For more than half of American adults who did not seek eye care, the reasons were cost or lack of awareness. The cost is often higher due to the lack of adequate health insurance. Among adults at high risk for vision loss, about 40 percent did not receive an eye exam in the last year. In 2017, approximately, 93 million U.S. adults aged 18 years or older, or about 4 in 10, were at high risk for vision loss. Among adults who reported needing eyeglasses, more than 8 million, or about 1 in 11, said they could not afford them. Data from the National Health Interview Survey, a nationally representative survey of noninstitutionalized civilians, were analyzed for this study. The analysis included nearly 33,000 survey respondents aged 18 or older in 2017, excluding adults who were blind or otherwise unable to see. Adults at high risk for vision loss included those who self-reported diagnosed diabetes, had vision and eye problems, or were 65 years or older.

These results suggest that improvements in eye care and affordable options for eyeglasses may prevent unnecessary vision loss. Annual eye exams are an important preventive care practice for people with diabetes. Early detection and treatment of diabetes-related eye disease and other eye diseases can prevent irreversible vision loss.[1]

SOCIAL DETERMINANTS AND HEALTH EQUITY

Social factors, such as where someone lives and their income level, can affect health outcomes, including the risk of vision loss. Social

---

[1] "Fast Facts: Vision Loss," Centers for Disease Control and Prevention (CDC), May 15, 2024. Available online. URL: www.cdc.gov/vision-health/data-research/vision-loss-facts/index.html. Accessed August 3, 2024.

determinants are key drivers of health inequities, particularly among people from racial and ethnic minority groups. Health inequities increase the risk of poor health outcomes, making it essential to reduce and eliminate these disparities to achieve health equity.

Social Determinants of Health and Vision Loss

Social determinants of health (SDOH) are nonmedical conditions that shape people's daily lives and influence their health, including where people live, learn, work, and play. Healthy People 2030 breaks SDOH into five key domains: education, health-care access, economic stability, built environment, and social context.

How Social Determinants Affect Vision Health

Income

People with lower incomes are less likely to access preventive care, such as eye exams, and more likely to have vision loss due to conditions like diabetic retinopathy (DR).

Education

Individuals with less than a high school education are less likely to have had an eye care visit in the past year compared to those with more education.

Neighborhood

Neighborhood safety can affect physical activity, weight management, blood sugar levels, and stress—all factors affecting diabetes risk and, consequently, vision loss.

Health-Care Access

People with vision impairments or blindness often report greater difficulties accessing care, citing issues such as cost, insurance coverage, transportation, and service refusal by providers. They are also more likely to be uninsured compared to those without vision impairment.[2]

---

[2] "Advancing Health Equity: Social Determinants and Vision Loss," Centers for Disease Control and Prevention (CDC), May 15, 2024. Available online. URL: www.cdc.gov/vision-health/health-equity/index.html. Accessed August 5, 2024.

Chapter 6 | Vision Loss: A Public Health Problem

Over 3.4 million Americans aged 40 years and older are blind or visually impaired, with this number expected to double by 2030. Vision loss reduces quality of life (QOL) and increases both direct and indirect costs. Early detection and treatment can prevent blindness and vision impairment.

Jinan B. Saaddine, a medical epidemiologist at the Centers for Disease Control and Prevention (CDC), along with coworkers, proposed five criteria to determine whether vision loss is a public health problem. These criteria are discussed below.

FIVE CRITERIA TO DEFINE A PUBLIC HEALTH PROBLEM

Does Vision Loss Affect Many People?

Yes. More than 3.4 million Americans aged 40 years and older are blind or visually impaired. Other estimates of vision problems go as high as 21 million people. Additionally, about 80 million Americans have diseases that can cause blindness.

Does Vision Loss Contribute to Poor Health and High Health-Care Costs?

Yes. People with vision loss are more likely to report having depression, diabetes, hearing impairment, stroke, falls, and cognitive decline. Those with vision loss are also more likely to die prematurely.

In addition, vision loss can make it difficult or impossible to drive, read, keep accounts, and navigate new places. These all contribute to a reduced QOL.

The economic burden of vision loss among Americans older than 40 years, including direct costs and lost productivity, is estimated to exceed $35 billion per year in the United States.

Has Vision Loss Recently Increased, and Will It Increase in the Future?

Yes. As the population of older people increases, the number of people with vision loss also rises. In addition, increases in the number of people with diabetes and other chronic conditions that can lead to eye diseases contribute to the rise in vision loss.

Prevent Blindness America estimates that the number of people with blindness and visual impairment will double by 2030 unless actions to prevent and treat eye diseases are taken.

Does the Public See Vision Loss as a Threat?

Yes. Many people fear vision loss due to its effect on QOL, daily activities, and independence.

Can Vision Loss Be Improved with Community or Public Health Action?

Yes. Research shows that early detection and treatment can prevent blindness and vision impairment. Screening and treatment for common eye conditions, such as diabetic retinopathy (DR), cataracts, and glaucoma, are available. However, many people are not screened, diagnosed, or treated.

For example, untreated age-related cataracts are a major cause of blindness among African-American people. Glaucoma is also still the leading blinding disease among African-American people, even though early detection and treatment can prevent vision loss.

Public health actions help to expand access to prevention and treatment for vision loss. Efforts also include population-based studies to identify trends in vision loss and which populations are most affected.[1]

[1] "Why Vision Loss Is a Public Health Problem," Centers for Disease Control and Prevention (CDC), May 15, 2024. Available online. URL: www.cdc.gov/vision-health/about-eye-disorders/vision-loss-public-health-problem.html. Accessed August 3, 2024.

Chapter 7 | Vision Impairment and Fall Prevention in Older Adults

Millions of Americans over 40 have vision impairment, and the number is increasing as the population ages. Each year, one in four Americans over 65 experience a fall, the leading cause of injury among older adults. Falls can often be prevented by protecting vision.

KNOW THE RISK

Older adults with impaired vision or who are at risk for vision impairment often have other chronic conditions. These may include diabetes, stroke, and heart disease, which also increase the risk of falling. In addition, some medicines taken for these conditions have side effects such as dizziness and muscle weakness, which can increase fall risk.

Older adults with vision impairment can also be socially isolated. They may take on physical tasks they cannot easily perform alone, increasing the risk of falls and injury. They may also have trouble getting help if they do fall.

PREVENTING FALLS

Falling and vision impairment are among the most common fears for older adults, but they can be prevented. You can reduce your risk by following these prevention strategies and slowing the progression of vision impairment.

- **Do exercises.** Improve your strength and balance, such as yoga, tai chi, or strengthening exercises.
- **Wear sturdy, nonslip footwear.** Choose shoes that fit correctly to help with balance and mobility.

- **Get a dilated eye exam at least once a year**. This reduces the risk of irreversible vision loss and ensures your prescription is up-to-date if you wear glasses.
- **Talk to your doctor**. Discuss evaluating your risk for vision impairment and falls. Ask if any of your medicines could cause side effects, such as drowsiness or dizziness, that increase your fall risk.
- **Make your home safer**:
    - Remove throw rugs or use double-sided tape to keep them from causing you to slip or trip.
    - Ensure good lighting in all rooms and hallways, with easily accessible switches or motion sensor lights.
    - Install handrails and grab bars on the stairs and in the bathroom/shower.

These steps can help older adults maintain their independence and reduce the risk of falls and injuries.[1]

[1] "About Vision Impairment and Falls among Older Adults," Centers for Disease Control and Prevention (CDC), May 15, 2024. Available online. URL: www.cdc.gov/vision-health/prevention/older-adult-falls.html. Accessed August 3, 2024.

Chapter 8 | Vision Loss and Mental Health

Over 7 million people in the United States experience vision loss, with many more at risk for severe vision impairment due to aging and chronic health conditions. As the U.S. population ages and the prevalence of chronic conditions increases, understanding the effect of vision loss on mental health and ways to maintain both eye and mental health becomes crucial.

VISION LOSS, DEPRESSION, AND ANXIETY

Vision loss can significantly affect physical health, quality of life (QOL), and mental well-being. It has been linked to loneliness, social isolation, and heightened feelings of worry, anxiety, and fear. Depression is particularly common among individuals with vision loss. A recent Centers for Disease Control and Prevention (CDC) study found that one in four adults with vision loss reported experiencing anxiety or depression. Notably, younger adults with vision loss are nearly five times more likely to experience severe anxiety or depression compared to older adults.

Untreated anxiety can increase the risk of developing depression. Therefore, it is essential for individuals with vision loss to be screened for these conditions. Early treatment can significantly improve the QOL.

SYMPTOMS OF DEPRESSION AND ANXIETY

If you experience symptoms of anxiety or depression, it is important to talk with your doctor. You may also seek a referral to a mental health counselor.

Common symptoms of anxiety include:

- trouble controlling feelings of worry
- difficulty focusing
- trouble sleeping
- feeling restless or on edge
- irritability

Common symptoms of depression include:

- lack of interest in hobbies and activities
- frequent feelings of sadness or anxiety
- feelings of helplessness or worthlessness
- changes in appetite and/or weight
- fatigue or lack of energy

TIPS FOR HEALTHY EYES AND A HEALTHY MIND

- **Add movement to your day**. Physical activity lowers your risk of developing health problems and can also boost your mood and reduce stress.
- **Eat healthy**. Nutritious food can improve your mood and lower your risk of type 2 diabetes and diabetic retinopathy (DR), one of the leading causes of vision loss.
- **Talk with your doctor about your family history**. Both mental health disorders and eye diseases can run in families.
- **Do not smoke**. People with mental health problems have a higher risk of serious health issues, often from smoking-related illnesses. Smoking also increases the risk of developing eye diseases that can cause vision loss.
- **Manage your chronic conditions**. Long-term health conditions such as cancer, heart disease, and diabetes may increase your chance of developing a mental health problem. Take your medications as prescribed and follow recommended lifestyle changes to help manage your health.

Vision loss can significantly affect both physical and mental health, but there are steps you can take to manage and improve your overall well-being. By staying active, eating well, and managing chronic conditions, you can maintain healthy eyes and a healthy mind. Additionally, seeking support for anxiety or depression can greatly enhance the QOL.[1]

[1] "About Vision Loss and Mental Health," Centers for Disease Control and Prevention (CDC), May 15, 2024. Available online. URL: www.cdc.gov/vision-health/about-eye-disorders/vision-loss-mental-health.html. Accessed August 3, 2024.

Part 2 | **Conditions Leading to Visual Impairment**

Chapter 9 | **Refractive Disorders**

Chapter Contents

Section 9.1 | Myopia (Nearsightedness)

WHAT IS NEARSIGHTEDNESS?

Nearsightedness is a refractive error that makes far-away objects look blurry. It occurs when the shape of the eye causes light to focus in front of the retina, a light-sensitive layer of tissue in the back of the eye, instead of directly on it. If you are nearsighted, your eye doctor can prescribe eyeglasses or contact lenses to help you see clearly.

WHAT CAUSES NEARSIGHTEDNESS?

Nearsightedness occurs when the eyeball grows too long from front to back, or when there are issues with the shape of the cornea (the clear front layer of the eye) or the lens (an inner part of the eye that helps focus light). These issues cause light to focus in front of the retina rather than on it, making far-away objects appear blurry.

WHAT ARE THE SYMPTOMS OF NEARSIGHTEDNESS?

The most common symptoms of nearsightedness include the following:

- trouble seeing things that are far away
- needing to squint to see clearly
- eye strain (when your eyes feel tired or sore)

Some people who are nearsighted may experience headaches, although this is less common. If you have mild nearsightedness, you may not notice any symptoms. Regular eye exams are important to ensure you see as clearly as possible.

People with severe nearsightedness (also called "high myopia") may also be at higher risk for other eye conditions, such as retinal detachment (when the retina is pulled away from its normal position).

ARE YOU AT RISK FOR NEARSIGHTEDNESS?

Anyone can develop nearsightedness, but you are at a higher risk if you have family members who are also nearsighted. Nearsightedness typically begins between ages 6 and 14 and worsens until the early twenties. Children who spend more time outdoors are less likely to become nearsighted, although the reason for this is not fully understood.

HOW WILL YOUR EYE DOCTOR CHECK FOR NEARSIGHTEDNESS?

Eye doctors can diagnose nearsightedness as part of a comprehensive eye exam. The exam is simple and painless.

WHAT IS THE TREATMENT FOR NEARSIGHTEDNESS?

The most common treatments for nearsightedness are eyeglasses or contact lenses. Your eye doctor will prescribe the appropriate lenses to help you see as clearly as possible. Adults may also opt for surgery to treat nearsightedness. The surgery involves reshaping the cornea to focus light correctly.[1]

Section 9.2 | Hyperopia (Farsightedness)

WHAT IS FARSIGHTEDNESS?

Farsightedness is a refractive error that makes nearby objects appear blurry. It occurs when the shape of the eye causes light to focus behind the retina, a light-sensitive layer of tissue at the back of the eye, instead of directly on it.

WHAT ARE THE SYMPTOMS OF FARSIGHTEDNESS?

The most common symptoms of farsightedness are:

- trouble seeing things up close
- eye strain (when your eyes feel tired or sore)
- headaches—especially when reading

If you have mild farsightedness, you may not notice any symptoms. Regular eye exams are important to ensure you see as clearly as possible.

Children with severe farsightedness may also be at higher risk for other eye problems, such as crossed eyes or amblyopia (lazy eye).

[1] "Nearsightedness," National Eye Institute (NEI), November 15, 2023. Available online. URL: www.nei.nih.gov/learn-about-eye-health/eye-conditions-and-diseases/nearsightedness-myopia. Accessed August 3, 2024.

WHAT CAUSES FARSIGHTEDNESS?

Farsightedness occurs when the eyeball grows too short from front to back, or when there are issues with the shape of the cornea (the clear front layer of the eye) or lens (an inner part of the eye that helps the eye focus). These issues cause light to focus behind the retina, making nearby objects appear blurry.

Most people who are farsighted are born with it, but it may not cause vision problems until later in life. You are more likely to be farsighted if other family members are also farsighted.

HOW WILL YOUR EYE DOCTOR CHECK FOR FARSIGHTEDNESS?

Eye doctors can diagnose farsightedness as part of a comprehensive eye exam. The exam is simple and painless.

WHAT IS THE TREATMENT FOR FARSIGHTEDNESS?

The most common treatments for farsightedness are eyeglasses or contact lenses. Your eye doctor will prescribe the appropriate lenses to help you see as clearly as possible.

Doctors can also use surgery to treat farsightedness in adults. The surgery changes the shape of the cornea so that it can focus light correctly.[1]

Section 9.3 | Astigmatism

WHAT IS ASTIGMATISM?

Astigmatism is a common eye condition that can cause blurry or distorted vision. It occurs when the cornea (the clear front layer of the eye) or lens (an inner part of the eye that helps focus light) has an irregular shape.

---

[1] "Farsightedness (Hyperopia)," National Eye Institute (NEI), November 15, 2023. Available online. URL: www.nei.nih.gov/learn-about-eye-health/eye-conditions-and-diseases/farsightedness-hyperopia. Accessed August 3, 2024.

WHAT CAUSES ASTIGMATISM?

Astigmatism is caused by an irregular shape of the cornea or lens, which causes light to bend unevenly as it enters the eye, leading to a refractive error. The exact cause of astigmatism is unknown, and there is no way to prevent it. Some people are born with astigmatism, while others develop it during childhood or early adulthood. It can also occur after an eye injury or surgery.

WHAT ARE THE SYMPTOMS OF ASTIGMATISM?

The most common symptoms of astigmatism include:

- blurry vision
- needing to squint to see clearly
- headaches
- eye strain
- trouble seeing at night

People with mild astigmatism may not notice any symptoms. Regular eye exams are important for detecting astigmatism and ensuring optimal vision, especially for children who may not realize their vision is impaired.

HOW WILL YOUR EYE DOCTOR CHECK FOR ASTIGMATISM?

Eye doctors can diagnose astigmatism during a comprehensive eye exam, which includes a dilated eye exam. The process is simple and painless.

WHAT IS THE TREATMENT FOR ASTIGMATISM?

The most common treatments for astigmatism include eyeglasses or contact lenses, which help correct vision. In some cases, surgery may be recommended to reshape the cornea, allowing it to focus light correctly.

If the astigmatism is mild, treatment may not be necessary. Your eye doctor will help determine the best course of action based on the severity of your condition.[1]

---

[1] "Astigmatism," National Eye Institute (NEI), November 15, 2023. Available online. URL: www.nei.nih.gov/learn-about-eye-health/eye-conditions-and-diseases/astigmatism. Accessed August 3, 2024.

Section 9.4 | Presbyopia

WHAT IS PRESBYOPIA?

Presbyopia is a common refractive error that affects middle-aged and older adults, making it difficult to see nearby objects clearly. This condition occurs when the lens (an inner part of the eye responsible for focusing light) loses its flexibility, preventing it from focusing light correctly on the retina (a light-sensitive layer of tissue at the back of the eye).

WHAT CAUSES PRESBYOPIA?

As people age, the lens in the eye becomes harder and less flexible, reducing its ability to focus light properly on the retina. This results in blurred vision for close objects. Presbyopia is distinct from farsightedness, another refractive error affecting near vision.

WHAT ARE THE SYMPTOMS OF PRESBYOPIA?

Common symptoms of presbyopia include:

- trouble seeing things up close
- needing to hold reading materials farther away to focus
- eye strain (tired or sore eyes)
- headaches

Presbyopia generally worsens over time but typically stabilizes after age 65.

HOW WILL YOUR EYE DOCTOR CHECK FOR PRESBYOPIA?

Eye doctors can diagnose presbyopia during a comprehensive eye exam, which is both simple and painless.

WHAT IS THE TREATMENT FOR PRESBYOPIA?

In the early stages of presbyopia, simple adjustments can help, such as:

- holding reading materials farther away
- choosing large-print books or increasing font size on digital devices
- using brighter reading lights

As presbyopia progresses, most people will need glasses or contact lenses to assist with reading. Some may use over-the-counter (OTC) reading glasses, while others may require prescription lenses from an eye doctor to achieve the best possible vision correction.[1]

Section 9.5 | Amblyopia (Lazy Eye)

WHAT IS AMBLYOPIA?

Amblyopia (also called "lazy eye") is a type of poor vision that usually happens in just one eye but less commonly in both eyes. It develops when there is a breakdown in how the brain and the eye work together, and the brain cannot recognize the sight from one eye. Over time, the brain relies more and more on the other, stronger eye—while vision in the weaker eye gets worse.

It is called "lazy eye" because the stronger eye works better. But people with amblyopia are not lazy, and they cannot control the way their eyes work. Amblyopia starts in childhood, and it is the most common cause of vision loss in kids. Up to 3 out of 100 children have it. The good news is that early treatment works well and usually prevents long-term vision problems.

WHAT CAUSES AMBLYOPIA?

In many cases, doctors do not know the cause of amblyopia. But sometimes, a different vision problem can lead to amblyopia. Normally, the brain uses nerve signals from both eyes to see. But if an eye condition makes vision in one eye worse, the brain may try to work around it. It starts to "turn off" signals from the weaker eye and rely only on the stronger eye.

Some eye conditions that can lead to amblyopia are:

- **Refractive errors**. These include common vision problems such as nearsightedness (having trouble seeing far away), farsightedness (having trouble seeing things up

---

[1] "Presbyopia," National Eye Institute (NEI), November 15, 2023. Available online. URL: www.nei.nih.gov/learn-about-eye-health/eye-conditions-and-diseases/presbyopia. Accessed August 3, 2024.

close), and astigmatism (which can cause blurry vision). Normally, these problems are easy to fix with glasses or contacts. But if they are not treated, the brain may start to rely more on the eye with stronger vision.
- **Strabismus**. Usually, the eyes move together as a pair. But in kids with strabismus, the eyes do not line up. One eye might drift in, out, up, or down.
- **Cataract**. This causes cloudiness in the lens of the eye, making things look blurry. While most cataracts happen in older people, babies and children can also develop cataracts.

WHAT ARE THE SYMPTOMS OF AMBLYOPIA?

Symptoms of amblyopia can be hard to notice. Kids with amblyopia may have poor depth perception—they have trouble telling how near or far something is. Parents may also notice signs that their child is struggling to see clearly, such as the following:
- squinting
- shutting one eye
- tilting their head

In many cases, parents do not know their child has amblyopia until a doctor diagnoses it during an eye exam. That is why it is important for all kids to get a vision screening at least once between ages three and five.

IS YOUR CHILD AT RISK FOR AMBLYOPIA?

Some kids are born with amblyopia and others develop it later in childhood. The chances of having amblyopia are higher in kids who:
- were born early (premature)
- were smaller than average at birth
- have a family history of amblyopia, childhood cataracts, or other eye conditions
- have developmental disabilities

HOW WILL YOUR CHILD'S DOCTOR CHECK FOR AMBLYOPIA?

As part of a normal vision screening, your child's doctor will look for signs of amblyopia. All kids aged three to five need to have their vision checked at least once.

WHAT IS THE TREATMENT FOR AMBLYOPIA?

If there is a vision problem causing amblyopia, the doctor may treat that first. For example, doctors may recommend glasses or contacts (for kids who are nearsighted or farsighted) or surgery (for kids with cataract).

The next step is to retrain the brain and force it to use the weaker eye. The more the brain uses it, the stronger it gets. Treatments include the following:

- **Wearing an eye patch on the stronger eye.** By covering up this eye with a stick-on eye patch (similar to a Band-Aid), the brain has to use the weaker eye to see. Some kids only need to wear the patch for two hours a day, while others may need to wear it whenever they are awake.
- **Putting special eye drops in the stronger eye.** A once-a-day drop of the drug atropine can temporarily blur near vision, which forces the brain to use the other eye. For some kids, this treatment works as well as an eye patch, and some parents find it easier to use (e.g., because young children may try to pull off eye patches).

After your child starts treatment, their vision may start to get better within a few weeks. But it will probably take months to get the best results. After that, your child may still need to use these treatments from time to time to stop amblyopia from coming back. It is important to start treating children with amblyopia early—the sooner, the better. Kids who grow up without treatment may have lifelong vision problems. Amblyopia treatment is usually less effective in adults than in children.[1]

[1] "Amblyopia (Lazy Eye)," National Eye Institute (NEI), September 22, 2022. Available online. URL: www.nei.nih.gov/learn-about-eye-health/eye-conditions-and-diseases/amblyopia-lazy-eye. Accessed May 2, 2024.

Section 9.6 | Keratoconus

WHAT IS KERATOCONUS?

Keratoconus is an eye condition that affects the shape of the cornea, the clear outer covering of the eye. Other names for this condition are "bulging cornea" and "conical cornea." In this condition, the cornea thins and bulges outward, eventually resembling a cone shape. These corneal abnormalities, which worsen over time, can lead to nearsightedness (myopia), blurred vision that cannot be improved with corrective lenses (irregular astigmatism), and vision loss.

Other corneal changes typical of keratoconus that can be seen during an eye exam include iron deposits in the cornea that form a yellow-to-brownish ring, called the "Fleischer ring," surrounding the colored part of the eye (iris). Affected individuals may also develop Vogt striae, which are thin, vertical, white lines in the tissue at the back of the cornea.

Keratoconus may affect only one eye at first, but eventually, the corneas of both eyes become misshapen, although they might not be affected with the same severity. As keratoconus worsens, people with this condition can develop corneal scarring, often caused by exposure of the abnormally thin cornea to prolonged contact lens use or excessive eye rubbing.

The eye changes characteristic of keratoconus typically begin in adolescence and slowly worsen until mid-adulthood, at which point the shape of the cornea remains stable.

FREQUENCY OF KERATOCONUS

Keratoconus is estimated to affect approximately 1 in 500–2,000 individuals worldwide.

CAUSES OF KERATOCONUS

The cause of keratoconus is unknown. Researchers have studied many different factors, both genetic and environmental, that are thought to influence the risk of developing keratoconus.

Environmental Factors

The environmental factors that may contribute to keratoconus include excessive eye rubbing and the tendency to develop allergic disorders (atopy).

Excessive and vigorous eye rubbing can cause trauma to the cornea and may lead to its thinning. However, it is unclear whether eye rubbing leads to keratoconus or if it is a response to eye discomfort in the early stages of the condition. If eye rubbing is not involved in the development of keratoconus, it likely contributes to its worsening.

Approximately one-third of individuals with keratoconus have an allergic disorder, although it is unclear how allergic disorders are related to the development of keratoconus. Allergies might trigger eye rubbing, which can aggravate eye problems.

Genetic Factors

Changes in multiple genes have been associated with developing keratoconus. Many of these variants have been found only in small populations or single families. In most individuals with keratoconus, a combination of genetic and environmental factors is necessary for the condition to develop. However, some affected individuals seem to have a largely environmental cause for the condition, while others seem to have a largely genetic cause. Individuals with a relative who has keratoconus have an increased risk of developing the condition compared to people without a family history.

More than a dozen genes have been associated with keratoconus. These genes have varied functions. The most frequently associated genes play roles in eye development, the formation and structure of the cornea, the intricate lattice of proteins and other molecules that forms in the space between cells (extracellular matrix), an immune system response called "inflammation," and the regulation of cell growth. It is thought that a disruption in one of these processes, in combination with an environmental trigger, may lead to the development of keratoconus.

Association with Genetic Syndromes

Keratoconus can be a feature of genetic syndromes, such as Leber congenital amaurosis and arterial tortuosity syndrome. When it is part of a syndrome, keratoconus is caused by the same genetic mutation that causes the syndrome. Mutations in the genes that cause syndromes with keratoconus have not been found to cause keratoconus without other features.

INHERITANCE OF KERATOCONUS

In most cases, keratoconus is not inherited and occurs in individuals with no family history of the disorder. The condition can also occur in families. In some cases, keratoconus is inherited in an autosomal dominant pattern, which means one copy of the altered gene in each cell is sufficient to cause the disorder. An affected person often has one parent with the condition, although some people who have a gene variant never develop the condition, a situation known as "reduced penetrance."

Keratoconus can also be inherited in an autosomal recessive pattern, which means variants occur in both copies of the gene in each cell. The parents of an individual with an autosomal recessive condition each carry one copy of the altered gene, but they typically do not show signs and symptoms of the condition.[1]

[1] MedlinePlus, "Refractive Errors," National Institutes of Health (NIH), July 1, 2017. Available online. URL: https://medlineplus.gov/genetics/condition/keratoconus/#synonyms. Accessed August 3, 2024.

Chapter 10 | **Cataracts**

Chapter Contents

Section 10.1 | How Cataracts Cloud Your Vision

As we age, our vision changes, and cataracts are a common change that affects many individuals. A cataract is a cloudy area in the lens of your eye. By age 80, most people either have cataracts or have had surgery to remove them.

THE DEVELOPMENT OF CATARACTS

Around age 40, the proteins in the lens of your eye start to break down and clump together. This clumping forms a cloudy area on your lens that worsens over time.

At first, you may not have any symptoms. However, eventually, your vision becomes blurry, and colors seem faded. You may also have trouble seeing at night.

CATARACT SURGERY

Luckily, cataracts can be corrected with surgery. Cataract surgery is one of the most common operations in the United States. Your doctor may recommend surgery if your cataracts begin to interfere with everyday activities such as reading, driving, or watching TV.

During cataract surgery, the doctor removes the clouded lens and replaces it with a new, artificial lens. Surgery is very safe. Nine out of ten people who undergo the procedure see better afterward. However, most people do not need to rush into surgery. Talk with your health-care provider if you are having vision problems.

PREVENTING AND DELAYING CATARACTS

There are several things you can do to delay the onset of cataracts:

- **Wear sunglasses and a hat**. These items help block the sun's harmful rays.
- **Quit smoking**. Smoking can accelerate the development of cataracts.
- **Eat a healthy diet**. Consume plenty of fruits and vegetables, especially dark, leafy greens like spinach and kale.

- **Regular eye exams.** If you are 60 years or older, get a dilated eye exam at least once every two years.[1]

Section 10.2 | Understanding and Managing Cataracts

WHAT ARE CATARACTS?

A cataract is a cloudy area in the lens of your eye. Cataracts are very common as you age. In fact, more than half of all Americans aged 80 or older either have cataracts or have had surgery to remove them.

At first, you may not notice that you have a cataract. But, over time, cataracts can make your vision blurry, hazy, or less colorful. You may have trouble reading or doing other everyday activities.

The good news is that surgery can remove cataracts. Cataract surgery is safe and corrects vision problems caused by cataracts.

WHAT CAUSES CATARACTS?

Most cataracts are caused by normal changes in the eyes as you age. When you are young, the lens in your eye is clear. Around age 40, the proteins in the lens start to break down and clump together. This clump forms a cloudy area on your lens—or a cataract. Over time, the cataract gets more severe and clouds more of the lens.

WHAT ARE THE SYMPTOMS OF CATARACTS?

You might not have any symptoms at first when cataracts are mild. But as they grow, cataracts can cause changes in your vision. For example, you may notice the following:

- Your vision is cloudy or blurry.
- The colors look faded.

[1] *NIH News in Health*, "How Cataracts Cloud Your Vision," National Institutes of Health (NIH), June 2020. Available online. URL: https://newsinhealth.nih.gov/2020/06/how-cataracts-cloud-your-vision. Accessed August 8, 2024.

- You cannot see well at night.
- Lamps, sunlight, or headlights seem too bright.
- You see a halo around the lights.
- You see double (this sometimes goes away as the cataract gets bigger).
- You must change the prescription for your glasses or contact lenses often.

Talk with your eye doctor if you have any of these symptoms—they could also be signs of other eye problems.

ARE YOU AT RISK FOR CATARACTS?

Your risk for cataracts goes up as you get older. You are also at higher risk if you:

- have certain health problems, such as diabetes
- are a smoker
- drink too much alcohol
- have a family history of cataracts
- have had an eye injury, eye surgery, or radiation treatment on your upper body
- have spent a lot of time in the sun
- take steroids (medicines used to treat a variety of health problems, such as arthritis and rashes)

If you are worried you might be at risk for cataracts, talk with your doctor. Ask if there is anything you can do to lower your risk.

HOW WILL YOUR EYE DOCTOR CHECK FOR CATARACTS?

An eye doctor can check for cataracts as part of a dilated eye exam. If you are 60 or older, get a dilated eye exam every one to two years. The exam is simple and painless—your doctor will give you some eye drops to dilate (widen) your pupil and then check your eyes for cataracts and other eye problems.

WHAT IS THE TREATMENT FOR CATARACTS?

Surgery is the only way to remove a cataract, but you may not need to get surgery right away.

- **Home treatment**. Early on, you may be able to make small changes to manage your cataracts. You can do things such as:
  - Use brighter lights at home or work.
  - Wear anti-glare sunglasses.
  - Use magnifying lenses for reading and other activities.
- **New glasses or contacts**. A new prescription for eyeglasses or contact lenses can help you see better with cataracts early on.
- **Surgery**. Your doctor might suggest surgery if your cataracts start getting in the way of everyday activities such as reading, driving, or watching TV. During cataract surgery, the doctor removes the clouded lens and replaces it with a new, artificial lens (also called an "intraocular lens" or "IOL"). This surgery is very safe, and 9 out of 10 people who get it can see better afterward.

Talk about your options with your doctor. Most people do not need to rush into surgery. Waiting to have surgery usually would not harm your eyes or make surgery more difficult later. Remember the following tips:

- Tell your doctor if cataracts are getting in the way of your everyday activities.
- See your doctor for regular checkups.
- Ask your doctor about the benefits and risks of cataract surgery.
- Encourage family members to get checked for cataracts since they can run in families.

HOW CAN YOU PREVENT CATARACTS?

You can take steps to protect your eyes from cataracts:

- **Protect your eyes from the sun**. Wear sunglasses and a hat with a brim to block the sun.
- **Protect your eyes from injury**. While doing activities such as using power tools or playing certain sports, wear protective eyewear to prevent eye injuries.

- **Quit smoking.** If you are ready to quit, call 800-QUIT-NOW (800-784-8669) for free support.
- **Make eye-healthy food choices.** Eat plenty of healthy foods—such as fruits and vegetables, leafy greens, nuts, and whole grains.[1]

Section 10.3 | Types of Cataracts

Most cataracts are age-related—they occur because of normal changes in your eyes as you age. However, cataracts can develop for other reasons, such as after an eye injury or surgery for another eye problem, such as glaucoma.

AGE-RELATED CATARACT

As you age, a cataract can develop due to natural changes in the lens of your eye. This is the most common type of cataract. You may be more likely to develop age-related cataracts if you:

- smoke
- drink excessive amounts of alcohol
- have a family history of cataracts
- have diabetes
- have undergone certain eye surgeries, such as glaucoma surgery
- take steroids—medicines used to treat some health problems, such as arthritis or allergies

TRAUMATIC CATARACT

Serious eye injuries can damage the lens and cause cataracts. The cataract may form quickly after the injury or develop many years later.

---

[1] "Cataracts," National Eye Institute (NEI), November 15, 2023. Available online. URL: www.nei.nih.gov/learn-about-eye-health/eye-conditions-and-diseases/cataracts. Accessed August 3, 2024.

RADIATION CATARACT

Certain types of radiation can cause cataracts. This includes ultraviolet (UV) rays from the sun and radiation treatment for cancer.

PEDIATRIC CATARACT

Children can also develop cataracts. They can be born with cataracts (congenital cataracts) or develop them later in life.

Cataracts in children are rare and are usually genetic—they tend to run in families. They can also occur due to serious complications during pregnancy or illnesses during childhood, such as uveitis or eye tumors. Children may also develop cataracts for the same reasons as adults—eye injuries, radiation, or steroid medications.

When pediatric cataracts are large enough to cause vision problems, they require immediate treatment. Early treatment is crucial to prevent other vision problems, such as amblyopia (lazy eye).

Other pediatric cataracts are so small that they may not affect your child's vision. Your child's doctor can monitor these smaller cataracts to ensure they do not cause vision issues.

SECONDARY CATARACT (POSTERIOR CAPSULE OPACIFICATION)

After cataract surgery, scar tissue can develop in the eye, clouding vision again. This condition is called a "secondary cataract." Other names for it include after-cataract or posterior capsule opacification. Secondary cataracts are common; in fact, up to two out of five people who have cataract surgery will develop a secondary cataract.

Treatment for secondary cataracts is quick and painless. Your eye doctor will use a laser to create an opening in the cloudy part of the lens—a procedure known as "YAG laser capsulotomy." Most people will notice their vision returning to normal within a few days.[1]

---

[1] "Types of Cataracts," National Eye Institute (NEI), January 4, 2023. Available online. URL: www.nei.nih.gov/learn-about-eye-health/eye-conditions-and-diseases/cataracts/types-cataract. Accessed August 3, 2024.

Chapter 11 | Retinal Diseases

Chapter Contents

Section 11.1 | Congenital Stationary Night Blindness

X-linked congenital stationary night blindness (XLCSNB) is a disorder of the retina. People with this condition typically experience night blindness and other vision problems, including loss of sharpness (reduced visual acuity), severe nearsightedness (myopia), nystagmus, and strabismus. Color vision is typically not affected. There are two major types of XLCSNB: the complete form and the incomplete form. Both types have very similar signs and symptoms. However, everyone with the complete form has night blindness, while not all people with the incomplete form have night blindness. The types are distinguished by their genetic causes.

WHAT CAUSES THIS DISEASE?

Congenital stationary night blindness is caused by genetic mutations, also known as "pathogenic variants." Genetic mutations can be hereditary when parents pass them down to their children, or they may occur randomly when cells are dividing. Genetic mutations may also result from contracted viruses, environmental factors such as ultraviolet (UV) radiation from sunlight exposure, or a combination of these.

If you suspect you may have this disease, you may want to start collecting your family health history. Information such as other family members who have had similar symptoms, when their/your symptoms first appeared, or exposures to any potential disease-causing environmental factors should be discussed with your medical team.

KNOWN GENETIC MUTATIONS

Genetic mutations in the following known genes cause congenital stationary night blindness:

- *CABP4*
- *PDE6B*
- *LRIT3*
- *CACNA1F*
- *GNAT1*
- *GNB3*
- *NYX*
- *GRM6*
- *SLC24A1*
- *TRPM1*
- *RHO*
- *GPR179*

Given these known genetic mutations, you may want to ask your health-care team if genetic testing is right for you. Genetic tests are laboratory tests that use samples of blood, saliva, or other tissues to help identify changes in genes, chromosomes, or proteins. Genetic testing can help confirm or rule out a suspected genetic disease or provide useful information to your health-care team.

SYMPTOMS

The types of symptoms experienced, and their intensity may vary among people with this disease. Your experience may be different from others. Consult your health-care team for more information.

The following are some symptoms associated with this disease:

- **Color vision defect**. An anomaly in the ability to discriminate between or recognize colors.
- **Compensatory head posture**. A compensatory head posture occurs when the head is deviated out of the normal primary straight head position to compensate for an ocular problem.
- **Electronegative electroretinogram**. A dark-adapted bright flash electroretinogram in which the b-wave is of markedly lower amplitude than the associated a-wave.
- **Hypermetropia**. An abnormality of refraction characterized by the ability to see objects in the distance clearly, while objects nearby appear blurry.
- **Myopia**. An abnormality of refraction characterized by the ability to see objects nearby clearly, while objects in the distance appear blurry.
- **Nyctalopia**. Inability to see well at night or in poor light.
- **Nystagmus**. Rhythmic, involuntary oscillations of one or both eyes related to an abnormality in fixation, conjugate gaze, or vestibular mechanisms.
- **Reduced amplitude of dark-adapted bright flash electroretinogram a-wave**. An abnormal reduction in the amplitude of the a-wave.

- **Retinal thinning**. Reduced anteroposterior thickness of the retina. This phenotype can be appreciated by retinal optical coherence tomography (OCT).
- **Strabismus**. A misalignment of the eyes so that the visual axes deviate from bifoveal fixation. The classification of strabismus may be based on several features, including the relative position of the eyes, whether the deviation is latent or manifest, intermittent or constant, concomitant or otherwise, and according to the age of onset and the relevance of any associated refractive error.

WHEN DO SYMPTOMS OF CONGENITAL STATIONARY NIGHT BLINDNESS BEGIN?

Symptoms of this disease may start to appear in a newborn.

CAN THIS DISEASE BE PASSED DOWN FROM PARENT TO CHILD?

Yes. It is possible for a biological parent to pass down genetic mutations that cause or increase the chances of getting this disease to their child. This is known as "inheritance." Knowing whether other family members have previously had this disease, also known as "family health history," can be very important information for your medical team.[1]

Section 11.2 | Retinopathy of Prematurity

WHAT IS RETINOPATHY OF PREMATURITY?

Retinopathy of prematurity (ROP) is an eye disease that can occur in babies who are premature (born early) or who weigh less than 3 pounds at birth. ROP happens when abnormal blood vessels grow in the retina, the light-sensitive layer of tissue at the back of the eye. Some babies with ROP have mild cases and improve without treatment, but others need treatment to protect their vision and prevent blindness.

---

[1] Genetic and Rare Diseases Information Center (GARD), "Congenital Stationary Night Blindness," National Center for Advancing Translational Sciences (NCATS), July 2024. Available online. URL: https://rarediseases.info.nih.gov/diseases/3995/congenital-stationary-night-blindness. Accessed August 3, 2024.

WHAT ARE THE STAGES OF RETINOPATHY OF PREMATURITY?

There are five stages of ROP, which doctors use to monitor the severity of the condition. These stages range from stage 1 (mild) to stage 5 (severe):

- **Stages 1 and 2**. Babies in these stages usually improve without treatment and go on to have healthy vision. Doctors monitor these babies closely to see if their ROP worsens.
- **Stage 3**. Some babies who develop stage 3 improve with no treatment and go on to have healthy vision. However, others need treatment to stop abnormal blood vessels from damaging the retina and causing retinal detachment, an eye condition that can lead to vision loss.
- **Stage 4**. Babies in stage 4 have partially detached retinas and require treatment.
- **Stage 5**. In stage 5, the retina detaches completely. Even with treatment, babies in stage 5 may experience vision loss or blindness.

Stages 4 and 5 are particularly serious, and babies in these stages often need surgery. However, even with treatment, they may experience vision loss. This is why doctors usually start treatment in stage 3.

It is also possible for babies in any stage to deteriorate quickly and need immediate treatment. Ensuring your baby receives their follow-up exams on schedule is crucial to lowering the risk of severe complications.

WHAT CAUSES RETINOPATHY OF PREMATURITY?

Normally, the blood vessels of the retina begin to develop in the fourth month of pregnancy and finish around the due date, or nine months of pregnancy. If a baby is born very early, these blood vessels may not develop normally. Instead, the retina may develop new, abnormal blood vessels, a process known as "retinal neovascularization" (NV). These abnormal vessels can grow in the wrong direction and, because they are attached to the retina, may pull the retina up off the back of the eye, leading to a type of retinal detachment.

WHAT ARE THE SYMPTOMS OF RETINOPATHY OF PREMATURITY?

Retinopathy of prematurity does not show visible signs. In advanced cases, the retina may partially or completely detach from its normal position, leading to retinal detachment, which can cause vision loss and blindness.

If your baby had ROP that caused damage, you may later notice that:

- **Their eyes wander, shake, or make other unusual movements**. Their eyes do not follow objects.
- **Their pupils appear white**. They have trouble recognizing faces.

Babies who had ROP are also more likely to develop other eye problems as they age, including:

- **Retinal detachment**. This condition can further impair vision.
- **Nearsightedness**. This can make distant objects appear blurry.
- **Amblyopia (lazy eye)**. This can result in decreased vision in one eye.
- **Crossed eyes**. This condition involves the eyes not aligning properly.

Regular checkups and eye exams are important for children who had ROP to help protect their vision as they grow.

IS YOUR BABY AT RISK FOR RETINOPATHY OF PREMATURITY?

Babies born before 30 weeks of pregnancy or weighing less than about 3 pounds are at risk for ROP. An eye specialist will check at-risk babies for ROP.

Babies are also more likely to develop ROP if they have:

- breathing problems and receive excessive oxygen therapy
- infections or other common premature medical issues, such as cardiac, pulmonary, or neurological problems

HOW WILL YOUR BABY'S DOCTOR CHECK FOR RETINOPATHY OF PREMATURITY?

At-risk babies typically undergo a dilated eye exam a few weeks after birth, usually between four and nine weeks. During the exam, the eye doctor will dilate your baby's pupils with eye drops and check every part of your baby's eye, especially the retina.

The need for follow-up exams depends on the initial findings. If necessary, the doctor will check your baby's eyes every one to three weeks until the risk for retinal detachment subsides.

WHAT IS THE TREATMENT FOR RETINOPATHY OF PREMATURITY?

Many babies with ROP improve without treatment. However, some require intervention to prevent the condition from worsening. Early treatment is crucial to protect your child's vision. Treatment options include:

- **Laser treatment**. For advanced ROP, laser treatment on the sides of the retina can prevent the condition from worsening and protect your child's vision.
- **Injections**. Doctors may inject anti-VEGF drugs into your baby's eye to block the growth of abnormal blood vessels.
- **Eye surgery**. For babies with partially or completely detached retinas (stages 4 or 5), options include:
    - **Scleral buckle surgery**. A flexible band is placed around the sclera to support the detached retina until normal growth resumes, after which the band is removed.
    - **Vitrectomy**. The doctor removes most of the vitreous and replaces it with saline solution, removes scar tissue from the retina, and may perform laser treatment to secure the retina.

Even with surgery, some babies with ROP will still experience vision loss or blindness.[1]

---

[1] "Retinopathy of Prematurity," National Eye Institute (NEI), November 15, 2023. Available online. URL: www.nei.nih.gov/learn-about-eye-health/eye-conditions-and-diseases/retinopathy-prematurity. Accessed August 3, 2024.

Section 11.3 | Retinoblastoma

Retinoblastoma is a disease in which malignant (cancer) cells form in the tissues of the retina. The retina is composed of nerve tissue that lines the inside wall of the back of the eye. It receives light and converts the light into signals that travel down the optic nerve to the brain.

Retinoblastoma may affect one eye (unilateral) or both eyes (bilateral). Cavitary retinoblastoma is a rare type of retinoblastoma in which cavities (hollow spaces) form within the tumor. Although retinoblastoma may occur at any age, it most often affects children younger than two.

Children with a family history of retinoblastoma should have eye exams to check for retinoblastoma. A child with a family history of retinoblastoma should have regular eye exams beginning early in life to check for retinoblastoma unless it is known that the child does not have the *RB1* gene change. Early diagnosis of retinoblastoma may mean the child will need less intense treatment. Discuss with your child's doctor the type of eye exam, how often eye exams are conducted, and at what age eye exams to check for retinoblastoma can stop.

SIGNS AND SYMPTOMS OF RETINOBLASTOMA

Signs and symptoms of retinoblastoma include a "white pupil" and eyes that appear to be looking in different directions (crossed eyes). These and other signs and symptoms may be caused by retinoblastoma or by other conditions. Consult with a doctor if your child exhibits any of the following:

- pupil of the eye appearing white instead of red when light shines into it (This may be observed in flash photographs of the child.)
- pain or redness in the eye
- infection around the eye
- eyeball that is larger than normal
- the colored part of the eye and pupil appearing cloudy

TESTS THAT EXAMINE THE RETINA ARE USED TO DIAGNOSE RETINOBLASTOMA

The following tests and procedures may be used:

- **Physical exam and health history**. An exam of the body to check general signs of health, including checking for signs of disease, such as lumps or anything else that seems unusual. A history of the patient's health habits and past illnesses and treatments will also be taken. The doctor will inquire if there is a family history of retinoblastoma.
- **Eye exam with dilated pupil**. This is an exam of the eye in which the pupil is dilated (opened wider) with medicated eye drops to allow the doctor to look through the lens and pupil to the retina. The inside of the eye, including the retina and the optic nerve, is examined with a light. In young children, this exam may be conducted under anesthesia.

There are several types of eye exams that are performed with the pupil dilated:

- ophthalmoscopy
- fluorescein angiography
- electroretinography
- *RB1* gene test
- ultrasound exam of the eye
- magnetic resonance imaging (MRI)

TREATMENT FOR RETINOBLASTOMA

Treatment for retinoblastoma depends on whether it is intraocular (within the eye) or extraocular (outside the eye).

- **Intraocular retinoblastoma**. In intraocular retinoblastoma, cancer is found in one or both eyes and may be in the retina only or in other parts of the eye, such as the choroid, ciliary body, or part of the optic nerve. Cancer has not spread to tissues around the outside of the eye or to other parts of the body.
- **Extraocular retinoblastoma (metastatic)**. In extraocular retinoblastoma, cancer has spread beyond the eye. It may be found in tissues around the eye (orbital retinoblastoma),

or it may have spread to the central nervous system (brain and spinal cord) or to other parts of the body such as the liver, bone, bone marrow, or lymph nodes.

Treatment for retinoblastoma also depends on whether the cancer has progressed or recurred. Progressive retinoblastoma is a cancer that continues to grow, spread, or get worse. Progressive disease may be a sign that the cancer has become refractory to treatment.

Recurrent retinoblastoma is a cancer that has recurred (come back) after it has been treated. The cancer may recur in the eye, in tissues around the eye, or in other places in the body, such as the liver, bone, bone marrow, or lymph nodes.

CERTAIN FACTORS AFFECT PROGNOSIS AND TREATMENT OPTIONS

The prognosis and treatment options depend on the following:

- whether the cancer is in one or both eyes
- the size and number of tumors
- whether the tumor has spread to the area around the eye, to the brain, or to other parts of the body
- the age of the child
- how likely it is that vision can be saved in one or both eyes
- whether a second type of cancer has formed
- whether the cancer is newly diagnosed or has recurred (come back)[1]

Section 11.4 | Retinitis Pigmentosa

WHAT IS RETINITIS PIGMENTOSA?

Retinitis pigmentosa (RP) is a group of rare eye diseases that affect the retina—the light-sensitive layer of tissue at the back of the eye. RP causes cells in the retina to break down slowly over time, leading

[1] "Retinoblastoma Treatment (PDQ®): Patient Version," National Cancer Institute (NCI), October 7, 2021. Available online. URL: www.cancer.gov/types/retinoblastoma/patient/retinoblastoma-treatment-pdq. Accessed August 3, 2024.

to vision loss. RP is a genetic disease that individuals are born with. Symptoms usually start in childhood, and most people eventually lose most of their sight.

WHAT CAUSES RETINITIS PIGMENTOSA?

Most commonly, RP is caused by changes in genes that control cells in the retina. These altered genes are inherited from parents to children. RP is associated with many different genes and can be inherited in various ways. If you have RP, you can consult with your doctor or a specialist known as a "genetic counselor" to learn more about your risk of passing RP to your children. Sometimes, RP occurs as part of other genetic conditions, such as Usher syndrome, which causes both vision and hearing loss.

WHAT ARE THE SYMPTOMS OF RETINITIS PIGMENTOSA?

The most common early symptom of RP is loss of night vision, usually starting in childhood. Parents may notice that children with RP struggle to navigate in the dark or to adjust to dim light. RP also causes loss of peripheral (side) vision, making it challenging to see objects out of the corners of your eyes. Over time, your field of vision narrows until you only have some central vision, also known as "tunnel vision." Some people with RP lose their vision more rapidly than others. Eventually, most individuals with RP lose both their side and central vision.

Other symptoms of RP include the following:

- sensitivity to bright light
- loss of color vision

HOW WILL YOUR EYE DOCTOR CHECK FOR RETINITIS PIGMENTOSA?

Eye doctors can check for RP as part of a comprehensive dilated eye exam. The exam is simple and painless. The doctor will administer eye drops to dilate (widen) your pupil and then examine your eyes for RP and other eye conditions. The exam also includes a visual field test to check peripheral (side) vision.

Other tests for RP include:

- **Electroretinography (ERG).** ERG allows the eye doctor to assess how well your retina responds to light.

- **Optical coherence tomography (OCT)**. This test uses light waves to take a detailed picture of your retina.
- **Fundus autofluorescence (FAF) imaging**. In this test, the eye doctor uses blue light to take a picture of the retina.
- **Genetic testing**. Your doctor may recommend a genetic test to learn more about the type of RP you have. This can inform you how your RP symptoms may change over time.

WHAT IS THE TREATMENT FOR RETINITIS PIGMENTOSA?

There is no cure for RP, but low vision aids and rehabilitation (training) programs can help people with RP make the most of their remaining vision. You can also discuss with your eye doctor the potential benefits of vitamins and supplements for RP. Vitamin A may help slow vision loss from the common forms of RP. However, taking too much vitamin A can cause liver problems—discuss the risks and benefits of this treatment with your doctor. Fish oil and lutein supplements may also help slow vision loss.

Early diagnosis and tailored interventions can significantly improve the quality of life (QOL) for those affected by this challenging condition.[1]

Section 11.5 | Diabetic Retinopathy

WHAT IS DIABETIC RETINOPATHY?

Diabetic retinopathy (DR) is an eye condition that can cause vision loss and blindness in individuals with diabetes. It affects the blood vessels in the retina, the light-sensitive layer of tissue at the back of your eye.

If you have diabetes, it is crucial to get a comprehensive dilated eye exam at least once a year. DR may not initially have any symptoms, but early detection can help you take steps to protect your vision.

---

[1] "Retinitis Pigmentosa," National Eye Institute (NEI), November 15, 2023. Available online. URL: www.nei.nih.gov/learn-about-eye-health/eye-conditions-and-diseases/retinitis-pigmentosa. Accessed August 3, 2024.

Managing your diabetes—by staying physically active, eating healthily, and taking your medication—can also help prevent or delay vision loss.

WHAT CAUSES DIABETIC RETINOPATHY?

Diabetic retinopathy is caused by high blood sugar levels due to diabetes. Over time, excessive sugar in your blood can damage your retina, the part of your eye that detects light and sends signals to your brain through the optic nerve.

Diabetes damages blood vessels throughout the body. The damage to your eyes begins when the sugar in your blood causes changes to the tiny blood vessels that supply your retina. These changes hinder blood flow, leading to blocked blood vessels that leak fluid or bleed. To compensate for these blocked vessels, your eyes then grow new blood vessels that do not function properly. These new vessels can leak or bleed easily.

WHAT OTHER PROBLEMS CAN DIABETIC RETINOPATHY CAUSE?

Diabetic retinopathy can lead to other serious eye conditions:

- **Diabetic macular edema (DME).** Over time, about half of the people with DR will develop DME. DME occurs when blood vessels in the retina leak fluid, causing swelling in the macula (a part of the retina). If you have DME, your vision will become blurry due to the excess fluid in your macula.
- **Neovascular glaucoma.** DR can cause abnormal blood vessels to grow out of the retina and block fluid from draining out of the eye, leading to a type of glaucoma.
- **Retinal detachment.** DR can cause scars to form at the back of the eye. When the scars pull the retina away from the back of the eye, it results in what is called "tractional retinal detachment."

WHAT ARE THE SYMPTOMS OF DIABETIC RETINOPATHY?

The early stages of DR typically do not have any symptoms. Some individuals notice changes in their vision, such as difficulty reading or seeing faraway objects. These changes may fluctuate.

In later stages of the disease, blood vessels in the retina begin to bleed into the vitreous, the gel-like fluid in the center of the eye. If this occurs, you may see dark, floating spots or streaks that resemble cobwebs. Sometimes, the spots clear up on their own, but it is crucial to seek treatment immediately. Without treatment, the bleeding can recur, worsen, or cause scarring.

ARE YOU AT RISK FOR DIABETIC RETINOPATHY?

Anyone with diabetes can develop DR, including individuals with type 1, type 2, and gestational diabetes (diabetes that can develop during pregnancy).

Your risk increases the longer you have diabetes. More than two in five Americans with diabetes have some stage of DR. Fortunately, you can lower your risk of developing DR by effectively managing your diabetes.

Women with diabetes who become pregnant or women who develop gestational diabetes are at high risk for developing DR. If you have diabetes and are pregnant, you should have a comprehensive dilated eye exam as soon as possible. Consult your doctor to determine if you will need additional eye exams during your pregnancy.

WHAT IS THE TREATMENT FOR DIABETIC RETINOPATHY AND DIABETIC MACULAR EDEMA?

In the early stages of DR, your eye doctor will likely monitor the condition of your eyes. Some individuals with DR may need a comprehensive dilated eye exam as often as every two to four months.

In later stages, it is crucial to begin treatment immediately—especially if you experience changes in your vision. While treatment cannot undo any damage to your vision, it can prevent your vision from worsening. It is also important to manage your diabetes, blood pressure, and cholesterol.

Treatments include:

- **Injections**. Medications called "anti-VEGF drugs" can slow down or reverse DR. Other medications, known as "corticosteroids," can also help.

- **Laser treatment.** To reduce swelling in your retina, eye doctors can use lasers to make the blood vessels shrink and stop leaking.
- **Eye surgery.** If your retina is bleeding significantly, or you have extensive scarring in your eye, your eye doctor may recommend a type of surgery known as "vitrectomy."

Having high blood pressure (HBP) or high cholesterol along with diabetes also increases your risk for DR. Therefore, controlling your blood pressure and cholesterol can help reduce your risk of vision loss.[1]

Section 11.6 | Diabetic Macular Edema

Diabetic macular edema (DME) affects the retina, particularly the macula, the central portion essential for clear vision. Elevated blood glucose levels damage the retina, causing fluid to leak from small blood vessels into the macula, resulting in swelling and vision distortion.

CAUSES OF DIABETIC MACULAR EDEMA

Diabetic macular edema commonly occurs in patients with diabetes mellitus, particularly diabetic retinopathy (DR), a condition that affects the retina's blood vessels. Multiple factors contribute to the development of DME:

- **Elevated blood glucose.** High blood glucose levels in the bloodstream cause DME, harming the retina's blood vessels.
- **Vascular endothelial growth factor (VEGF).** Overproduction of VEGF, a protein that increases vascular permeability, leads to inflammation and fluid leakage, contributing to DME.
- **Cholesterol.** High cholesterol levels may contribute to DME.

[1] "Diabetic Retinopathy," National Eye Institute (NEI), June 28, 2024. Available online. URL: www.nei.nih.gov/learn-about-eye-health/eye-conditions-and-diseases/diabetic-retinopathy. Accessed August 3, 2024.

- **Microvascular alteration.** Chronic high blood sugar levels can activate many metabolic pathways that lead to abnormalities in small blood vessels in the retina. These modifications involve weakening and dilatation of blood vessels, leakage of fluids, and vessel closure.
- **Ischemia.** Reduced blood flow to the retina, caused by obstructions in the retinal blood vessels, can worsen DME. Ischemia weakens the blood-retinal barrier, which causes the development of abnormal blood vessels that are likely to leak.
- **Advanced glycation end products (AGEs).** High glucose levels in diabetes can lead to the production of AGEs, which build up in the retinal blood vessels, causing vascular dysfunction and inflammation. AGEs also hinder the function of cells in the retina, increasing the progression of DME.

SIGNS AND SYMPTOMS OF DIABETIC MACULAR EDEMA

Diabetic macular edema commonly presents with various signs and symptoms. A few common indications include:

- **Blurry or distorted central vision.** Fluid accumulation in the macular structure can lead to blurred or distorted vision, leading to difficulty in perceiving fine details.
- **Reading difficulty.** Individuals with DME may struggle with reading tasks due to hazy or unclear vision.
- **Altered color perception.** DME can cause challenges in differentiating between colors or perceiving them appropriately. Colors may seem faded.
- **Central scotoma.** Some individuals with DME may experience a central scotoma, a blind spot or area of impaired vision that can affect activities requiring clear central vision, such as driving or watching television.
- **Floaters.** They are small, dark spots or specks that appear to float in the field of vision. These are not exclusive to DME, but changes in the vitreous humor may make them more noticeable in patients with DME.

DIAGNOSTIC PROCEDURE OF DIABETIC MACULAR EDEMA

The following methods are used to diagnose DME:

- **Evaluation of visual acuity**. Visual acuity is assessed, usually with standardized vision charts, to quantify the degree of DME-related vision impairment. Testing establishes initial data and aids in tracking alterations in eyesight over time.
- **Ophthalmoscopy**. Ophthalmologists dilate the eye to examine the fundus, the eye's posterior segment, including the optic nerve, retina, and macula. Using tools such as the slit lamp and ophthalmoscope, they can detect retinal hemorrhages, microaneurysms, hard exudates, and macular thickness.
- **Ocular coherence tomography (OCT)**. This noninvasive imaging technique offers high-resolution cross-sectional images of the retina and optic nerve, enabling a detailed view for assessing retinal layers and detecting macular edema.
- **Fluorescein angiography (FA)**. This procedure involves the intravenous injection of a fluorescent dye to assess the blood flow in the retina. FA can detect retinal ischemia, blood leakage, and abnormal blood vessel growth associated with DME.

TREATMENT OF DIABETIC MACULAR EDEMA

The various methods used to treat DME include:

- **Corticosteroid injections**. Corticosteroids such as fluocinolone, triamcinolone acetonide, or dexamethasone are injected into the eye to reduce inflammation and swelling.
- **Anti-VEGF**. Medications such as ranibizumab, aflibercept, and bevacizumab are administered through injection into the eye to bind to the VEGF. This aids in decreasing edema and enhancing vision.
- **Laser therapy**. Focal or grid laser photocoagulation treatment closes leaking blood vessels and decreases edema.

- **Surgery**. Vitrectomy surgery may be an option in some situations. During this treatment, vitreous gel and any scar tissue on the retina are extracted from the eye to enhance vision.

PREVENTION OF DIABETIC MACULAR EDEMA

Certain lifestyle changes that help prevent DME include:

- **Blood glucose level management**. It is crucial to maintain blood glucose levels through dietary management, physical activity, medication, and consistent monitoring. This aids in decreasing the likelihood and progression of DME.
- **Regular eye examinations**. Periodic eye examinations are essential for preventing and identifying DME. Timely medical intervention can prevent visual loss or slow its progression.
- **Smoking cessation**. Smoking increases the risk of DME and other health issues. Quitting smoking can lower the risk and slow down the progression of DME.
- **Monitoring vision changes**. Timely identification and management of DME-related vision changes can reduce the risk of vision impairment.

LIVING WITH DIABETIC MACULAR EDEMA

In time, DME can impair an individual's vision. Effective ways to manage DME include:

- **Low vision aids**. Using low-vision aids such as magnifying glasses, lenses, bright reading lamps, and telescopic lenses can help individuals with inadequate vision improve their remaining vision.
- **Occupational therapy (OT)**. Engaging in OT can help enhance the patient's ability to perform daily activities and tasks more efficiently.
- **Vision rehabilitation**. This includes mobility training, assistive technology, adaptive strategies for daily living, counseling, and support to help individuals live independently.

Early diagnosis and treatment are crucial to prevent permanent vision loss in the diabetic population.

References

"Diabetes-Related Macular Edema," Cleveland Clinic, February 14, 2023. Available online. URL: https://my.clevelandclinic.org/health/diseases/24733-diabetes-related-macular-edema. Accessed August 7, 2024.

"Diabetes-Related Macular Edema," Prevent Blindness, February 22, 2016. Available online. URL: https://preventblindness.org/diabetic-macular-edema-dme. Accessed August 7, 2024.

"Diabetic Macular Edema," Mayo Clinic, January 29, 2015. Available online. URL: www.mayoclinic.org/diseases-conditions/diabetic-retinopathy/multimedia/diabetic-macular-edema/img-20124558. Accessed August 7, 2024.

Key, Alyson Powell. "Lifestyle Changes for Diabetic Macular Edema," *Web*MD, December 6, 2023. Available online. URL: www.webmd.com/diabetes/lifestyle-changes-diabetic-macular-edema. Accessed August 7, 2024.

Pisacreta, Emily. "Tips for Managing Life with Diabetic Macular Edema," Healthline, February 8, 2023. Available online. URL: www.healthline.com/health/eye-health/tips-managing-diabetic-macular-edema. Accessed August 7, 2024.

Rath, Linda. "A Closer Look at Diabetic Macular Edema," *Web*MD, December 6, 2023. Available online. URL: www.webmd.com/diabetes/diabetic-macular-edema-causes-symptoms. Accessed August 7, 2024.

Rath Linda. "Treatments for Diabetic Macular Edema," *Web*MD, December 6, 2023. Available online. URL: www.webmd.com/diabetes/diabetic-macular-edema-treatment. Accessed August 7, 2024.

Stuart, Annie. "Diabetic Macular Edema," *Web*MD, April 11, 2023. Available online. URL: www.webmd.com/diabetes/diabetic-macular-edema#091e9c5e80fb6a53-1-3. Accessed August 7, 2024.

Werner, Carly. "Diabetic Macular Edema: What You Need to Know," Healthline, October 12, 2020. Available online. URL: www.healthline.com/health/eye-health/diabetic-macular-edema-symptoms-treatment. Accessed August 7, 2024.

Section 11.7 | Retinal Detachment

WHAT IS RETINAL DETACHMENT?

Retinal detachment is an eye condition that occurs when the retina—a light-sensitive layer of tissue at the back of your eye—is pulled away from its normal position at the back of your eye.

TYPES AND CAUSES OF RETINAL DETACHMENT

There are many causes of retinal detachment, but the most common are aging or an eye injury. There are three types of retinal detachment:

- rhegmatogenous
- tractional
- exudative

Each type results from a different issue that causes your retina to move away from the back of your eye. Any type of retinal detachment is a medical emergency. If you experience symptoms of a detached retina, seek immediate medical attention. Early treatment can help prevent permanent vision loss.

Rhegmatogenous Retinal Detachment

Rhegmatogenous retinal detachment is the most common type. It occurs if there is a small tear or break in your retina. When the retina tears, the vitreous—the gel-like fluid in the center of your eye—can seep behind the retina, pushing it away from the back of your eye and causing detachment. Aging is the primary cause of rhegmatogenous retinal detachment. As you age, the vitreous in your eye may change in texture and shrink. Occasionally, as it shrinks, it can tug on the retina and cause it to tear. Other factors that can increase your risk include eye injuries, eye surgeries, and nearsightedness.

Tractional Retinal Detachment

Tractional retinal detachment occurs if scar tissue on your retina pulls it away from the back of your eye. The most common cause of tractional retinal detachment is diabetic retinopathy (DR)—an eye condition that affects individuals with diabetes. DR damages the blood vessels in the retina and can cause scarring. As the scars worsen, they can pull on the retina, causing it to detach. It is crucial for individuals with diabetes to undergo comprehensive dilated eye exams annually. Managing your diabetes through physical activity, a healthy diet, and medication can also help prevent or delay vision loss. Other causes of tractional retinal detachment include eye diseases, infections, and swelling.

Exudative Retinal Detachment

Exudative retinal detachment occurs when fluid accumulates behind your retina without any tears or breaks in the retina itself. If enough fluid accumulates, it can push the retina away from the back of your eye, causing detachment. The most common causes of exudative retinal detachment are leaking blood vessels or swelling at the back of the eye, which can be due to:

- injury or trauma to the eye
- age-related macular degeneration (AMD)
- tumors in the eye
- diseases that cause inflammation inside the eye
- Coats disease, a rare eye disorder

WHAT ARE THE SYMPTOMS OF RETINAL DETACHMENT?

If only a small portion of your retina detaches, you might not notice any symptoms. However, if a larger area is affected, you may experience a significant decline in your ability to see clearly. Other sudden symptoms might include:

- numerous new floaters (small dark spots or squiggly lines that float across your vision)
- flashes of light in one or both eyes

- a dark shadow or "curtain" falling across the sides or middle of your field of vision

Since retinal detachment is a medical emergency, seek immediate care if you notice these symptoms. The symptoms often develop quickly, and without prompt treatment, more of the retina can detach, increasing the risk of permanent vision loss or blindness.

WHAT IS THE TREATMENT FOR RETINAL DETACHMENT?

The treatment for retinal detachment depends on the extent and type of detachment. Your eye doctor might recommend laser surgery, freezing treatment (cryopexy), or other surgical procedures to repair tears or breaks and reattach the retina.

- **Freeze treatment (cryopexy) or laser surgery**. For small holes or tears, these treatments can seal the retina and are usually performed in the doctor's office.
- **Surgery**. For larger detachments, you might need surgery in a hospital to reposition the retina.

Treatment is highly effective, especially if the detachment is diagnosed early. If the retina detaches again, a second treatment might be necessary, but about 90 percent of cases are successfully resolved with treatment.

HOW CAN YOU PREVENT RETINAL DETACHMENT?

While it is not possible to prevent retinal detachment entirely, you can reduce your risk by wearing safety goggles or other protective eyewear during high-risk activities. If you experience any symptoms of retinal detachment, seek immediate medical attention. Early treatment can help prevent permanent vision loss. Regular comprehensive dilated eye exams are also crucial, as they can detect retinal tears or detachments early before they significantly affect your vision.[1]

---

[1] "Retinal Detachment," National Eye Institute (NEI), November 15, 2023. Available online. URL: www.nei.nih.gov/learn-about-eye-health/eye-conditions-and-diseases/retinal-detachment. Accessed August 3, 2024.

Section 11.8 | Late-Onset Retinal Degeneration

WHAT IS LATE-ONSET RETINAL DEGENERATION?

Late-onset retinal degeneration is an inherited retinal dystrophy characterized by delayed dark adaptation, nyctalopia, and drusen deposits that present in adulthood. Cone and rod degeneration typically begins in the sixth decade of life, leading to central vision loss. The anterior segment features, such as peripapillary iris transillumination defects and abnormally long anterior zonular insertions, are also observed. In the late stages of the disease, choroidal neovascularization and glaucoma may occur.

WHAT CAUSES THIS DISEASE?

Late-onset retinal degeneration is caused by genetic mutations, also known as "pathogenic variants." These mutations can be hereditary, passed down from parents to their children, or they may occur spontaneously when cells divide. Additionally, genetic mutations may result from contracted viruses, environmental factors such as ultraviolet (UV) radiation from sunlight, or a combination of these factors.

SYMPTOMS

The types and intensity of symptoms can vary among individuals with this disease. Your experience may differ from that of others. For more information, consult your health-care team.

Symptoms associated with this condition include:

- **Abnormal anterior eye segment morphology**. Anomaly of the anterior segment of the eyeball, which includes the cornea, iris, ciliary body, and lens.
- **Abnormal suspensory ligament of lens morphology**. An anomaly of the suspensory ligament of the lens, also known as the "ciliary zonule," which holds the lens in place.
- **Chorioretinal atrophy**. Atrophy of the choroid and retinal layers of the fundus.
- **Choroidal neovascularization**. Formation of new blood vessels in the choroid layer of the eye.

- **Drusen**. Yellow or white accumulations of extracellular material in Bruch's membrane of the eye.
- **Epiretinal membrane**. A fibrous tissue that develops on the surface of the retina and can potentially disturb vision. It is also known as "macular pucker," "macular fibrosis," "surface wrinkling retinopathy," or "cellophane maculopathy."
- **Iris atrophy**. Loss of iris tissue.
- **Iris transillumination defect**. Light transmission through the iris visible during slit-lamp examination or infrared iris transillumination videography.
- **Macular atrophy**. Defined areas of partial or complete depigmentation in the macula, indicating loss of retinal pigment epithelium and photoreceptor cells.
- **Macular degeneration**. Degeneration of the retinal pigment epithelium and/or retinal photoreceptor cells in the macula lutea.
- **Multifocal subretinal deposits**. Deposits accumulating between the outer retina and the retinal pigment epithelium.
- **Nyctalopia**. Difficulty seeing in low light or at night.
- **Ocular hypertension**. Elevated intraocular pressure above the population mean.
- **Patchy atrophy of the retinal pigment epithelium**. Isolated areas of atrophy in the retinal pigment epithelium.
- **Peripapillary atrophy**. Thinning of the retina and retinal pigment epithelium around the optic nerve.
- **Photophobia**. Excessive sensitivity to light causing discomfort or pain.
- **Red-green dyschromatopsia**. Difficulty distinguishing red and green hues.
- **Severely reduced visual acuity**. A significant reduction in the ability to see, defined as visual acuity less than 6/60 (20/200 in US notation; 0.1 in decimal notation) but at least 3/60 (20/400 in US notation; 0.05 in decimal notation).

- **Tritanomaly**. Difficulty distinguishing between yellow and blue, possibly related to dysfunction of the S photopigment.
- **Visual loss**. A decrease in visual acuity from a previous point in life.

CAN THIS DISEASE BE PASSED DOWN FROM PARENT TO CHILD?

Yes, it is possible for a biological parent to pass down genetic mutations that cause or increase the chances of acquiring this disease to their child. This is known as "inheritance." Knowing whether other family members have had this disease, also known as "family health history," can be crucial information for your medical team.

Understanding the genetic basis and symptomatic presentation of late-onset retinal degeneration is essential for effective management and familial planning. Early diagnosis through genetic testing and regular monitoring can help manage symptoms and prevent progression.[1]

[1] Genetic and Rare Diseases Information Center (GARD), "Late-Onset Retinal Degeneration," National Center for Advancing Translational Sciences (NCATS), July 2024. Available online. URL: https://rarediseases.info.nih.gov/diseases/4357/late-onset-retinal-degeneration. Accessed August 3, 2024.

Chapter 12 | Glaucoma

WHAT IS GLAUCOMA?

Glaucoma is a group of eye diseases that can cause vision loss and blindness by damaging a nerve in the back of your eye called the "optic nerve."

The symptoms can start so slowly that you may not notice them. The only way to find out if you have glaucoma is to get a comprehensive dilated eye exam.

There is no cure for glaucoma, but early treatment can often stop the damage and protect your vision.

WHAT ARE THE TYPES OF GLAUCOMA?

When experts do not know what causes a type of glaucoma, that type is called a "primary glaucoma."

Open-angle glaucoma is the most common type in the United States, where 9 in 10 people with glaucoma have the open-angle type. Many people do not have any symptoms until they start to lose their vision, and people may not notice vision loss right away.

Other types are less common, such as:

- angle-closure glaucoma
- normal-tension glaucoma
- congenital glaucoma
- secondary glaucomas
- neovascular glaucoma
- pigmentary glaucoma
- exfoliation glaucoma (pseudoexfoliation)
- uveitic glaucoma

WHAT CAUSES GLAUCOMA?

Scientists are not sure what causes the most common types of glaucoma, but many people with glaucoma have high eye pressure (intra-ocular pressure)—and treatments that lower eye pressure help to slow the disease.

There is no way to prevent glaucoma. That is why eye exams are so important—so you and your doctor can find it before it affects your vision.

WHAT ARE THE SYMPTOMS OF GLAUCOMA?

At first, glaucoma does not usually have any symptoms. That is why half of the people with glaucoma do not even know they have it.

Over time, you may slowly lose vision, usually starting with your side (peripheral) vision—especially the part of your vision that is closest to your nose. Because it happens so slowly, many people cannot tell that their vision is changing, especially at first.

But, as the disease gets worse, you may start to notice that you cannot see things off to the side anymore. Without treatment, glaucoma can eventually cause blindness.

ARE YOU AT RISK FOR GLAUCOMA?

Anyone can get glaucoma, but some people are at higher risk. You are at higher risk if you:

- are over age 60, especially if you are Hispanic/Latino
- are African American and over age 40
- have a family history of glaucoma

Talk with your doctor about your risk for glaucoma, and ask how often you need to get checked. If you are at higher risk, you need to get a comprehensive dilated eye exam every one to two years.

WHAT IS THE TREATMENT FOR GLAUCOMA?

Doctors use a few different types of treatment for glaucoma, including medicines (usually eye drops), laser treatment, and surgery. If you have glaucoma, it is important to start treatment right away. While it will not undo any damage to your vision, treatment can stop it from worsening.

- **Medicines.** Prescription eye drops are the most common treatment. They lower the pressure in your eye and prevent damage to your optic nerve.

- **Laser treatment**. Doctors can use lasers to help fluid drain out of your eye to lower pressure. This is a simple procedure that your doctor can perform in the office.
- **Surgery**. If medicines and laser treatment do not work, your doctor might suggest surgery. Several types of surgery can help the fluid drain out of your eye.[1]

[1] "Glaucoma," National Eye Institute (NEI), November 15, 2023. Available online. URL: www.nei.nih.gov/learn-about-eye-health/eye-conditions-and-diseases/glaucoma. Accessed August 3, 2024.

Chapter 13 | **Macular Degeneration**

Chapter Contents

Section 13.1 | Age-Related Macular Degeneration

WHAT IS AGE-RELATED MACULAR DEGENERATION?

Age-related macular degeneration (AMD) is an eye disease that can blur central vision. It occurs when aging causes damage to the macula, the part of the eye that controls sharp, straight-ahead vision. The macula is part of the retina, the light-sensitive tissue at the back of the eye.

It is a common condition and a leading cause of vision loss for older adults. AMD does not cause complete blindness, but losing your central vision can make it harder to see faces, read, drive, or do close-up work such as cooking or fixing things around the house.

It progresses very slowly in some people and faster in others. Even if you have early AMD, you may not experience vision loss for a long time. Therefore, it is important to get regular eye exams to find out if you have AMD.

WHAT ARE THE TYPES AND STAGES OF AMD?

There are two types of AMD: Dry and Wet.

Most people with AMD have dry AMD (also called "atrophic AMD"). This type occurs when the macula gets thinner with age. Dry AMD happens in three stages: early, intermediate, and late. It usually progresses slowly over several years. There is no treatment for late dry AMD, but you can find ways to make the most of your remaining vision. And if you have late dry AMD in only one eye, you can take steps to protect your other eye.

Wet AMD (also called "advanced neovascular AMD") is a less common type of late AMD that usually causes faster vision loss. Any stage of dry AMD can turn into wet AMD—but wet AMD is always late stage. It happens when abnormal blood vessels grow in the back of the eye and damage the macula. The good news is that treatment options are available for wet AMD.

WHAT ARE THE SYMPTOMS OF AGE-RELATED MACULAR DEGENERATION?

The symptoms of AMD depend on the stage. Dry AMD occurs in three stages: early, intermediate, and late. AMD is a progressive disease—that means symptoms usually worsen over time.

Early dry AMD does not cause any symptoms.

In intermediate dry AMD, some people still have no symptoms. Others may notice mild symptoms, such as mild blurriness in their central vision or trouble seeing in low lighting.

In late AMD (wet or dry type), many people notice that straight lines start to look wavy or crooked. You may also notice a blurry area near the center of your vision. Over time, this blurry area may get bigger, or you may see blank spots. Colors may also seem less bright than before, and you may have more trouble seeing in low lighting.

Straight lines that look wavy are a warning sign for late AMD. If you notice this symptom, see your eye doctor right away.

ARE YOU AT RISK FOR AGE-RELATED MACULAR DEGENERATION?

Your risk for AMD increases as you get older. People aged 55 and older are more likely to have AMD. The risk for AMD is also higher for people who:

- have a family history of AMD
- are Caucasian
- smoke

If you are at risk for AMD because of your age, family history, or other factors, it is important to get regular eye exams. Ask your doctor how often you need to get eye exams. Early AMD does not have any symptoms, so do not wait for your vision to change.

HOW CAN YOU LOWER YOUR RISK FOR AGE-RELATED MACULAR DEGENERATION?

Research shows that you may be able to lower your risk of AMD (or slow its progression) by making these healthy choices:

- Quit smoking—or do not start.
- Get regular physical activity.
- Maintain healthy blood pressure and cholesterol levels.
- Eat healthy foods, including leafy green vegetables and fish.

WHAT IS THE TREATMENT FOR AGE-RELATED MACULAR DEGENERATION?

Treatment for AMD depends on the stage and type. There is currently no treatment for early AMD, so your eye doctor will probably just monitor your eyes with regular eye exams. Eating healthy, getting regular exercise, and quitting smoking can also help.

If you have intermediate AMD in one or both eyes, special dietary supplements (vitamins and minerals) may be able to stop it from turning into late AMD. If you have late AMD in only one eye, these supplements may slow down AMD in your other eye.

If you have wet AMD, there are other treatments that may be able to stop further vision loss:

- anti-vascular endothelial growth factor (VEGF) drugs that the doctor injects in your eye
- photodynamic therapy (PDT), a combination of injections and laser treatment

There is currently no treatment for late dry AMD, but researchers are hard at work finding treatment options. You can also get support to help you live with vision loss from AMD.

HOW DO YOU LIVE WITH VISION LOSS FROM AGE-RELATED MACULAR DEGENERATION?

Not everyone with AMD develops late AMD or experiences it in both eyes. However, if you do, living with vision loss from AMD can be challenging. Having low vision means that even with glasses, contact lenses, medicine, or surgery, your vision impairment makes it difficult to perform everyday tasks.

Fortunately, there are resources available that can help—such as low-vision devices and vision rehabilitation services. Vision rehabilitation can help you learn the skills you need to remain independent and active despite low vision.[1]

---

[1] "Age-Related Macular Degeneration (AMD)," National Eye Institute (NEI), June 22, 2021. Available online. URL: www.nei.nih.gov/learn-about-eye-health/eye-conditions-and-diseases/age-related-macular-degeneration. Accessed August 3, 2024.

Section 13.2 | Macular Hole

WHAT IS A MACULAR HOLE?

A macular hole is a rare eye condition that can blur the central vision you use for everyday tasks such as driving or reading.

The macula is a small area in the center of the retina (the light-sensitive layer of tissue in the back of the eye). Macular holes occur when an opening forms in the macula—usually after being stretched or pulled. Most macular holes form due to changes in the eye that occur as you age.

Some people with macular holes have mild symptoms and may not need treatment right away. However, if a macular hole is getting bigger, worsening, or causing serious vision problems, doctors may recommend surgery to protect vision.

WHAT CAUSES A MACULAR HOLE?

Most of the time, a macular hole occurs due to changes in your eye as you age.

As you age, the vitreous (the clear gel-like fluid that fills your eye and gives it a round shape) shrinks and pulls away from the retina. This is called "vitreous detachment," and it happens to everyone as they get older.

In some people, the vitreous is attached more firmly to the macula and pulls on it as it detaches. This pulling and stretching of the retina can cause a macular hole.

WHAT ARE THE SYMPTOMS OF A MACULAR HOLE?

If your other eye has good vision, you may not notice any symptoms from a macular hole. When a macular hole does cause symptoms, they often start slowly.

At first, you might notice that things look distorted or blurry when you look straight ahead. Lines or straight objects—such as a window frame—might appear bent, wavy, or missing a piece in the center. It might be harder to perform everyday tasks such as reading, writing, or driving.

Over time, you might notice a blurred or blind spot in your central vision. When reading, you may see the lines but miss letters or words in the center. Or you may be able to see a person's face but not their nose or eyes.

Early treatment with surgery can often restore vision. Without early treatment, central vision loss may be permanent.

IS A MACULAR HOLE THE SAME AS AGE-RELATED MACULAR DEGENERATION?

No. Macular holes and age-related macular degeneration can cause similar symptoms, and they are both common in people over age 60, but they are different conditions. If you are not sure which condition you have, talk to your eye doctor.

ARE YOU AT RISK FOR A MACULAR HOLE?

If you have previously had a macular hole in one eye, you are more likely to develop one in the other eye as well. About 1 in 10 people who get a macular hole in one eye will develop a macular hole in their other eye.

You are also at risk for a macular hole if you:

- are 60 years old or older
- are very nearsighted
- have had an eye injury or eye surgery

HOW WILL YOUR EYE DOCTOR CHECK FOR A MACULAR HOLE?

Your eye doctor will check for a macular hole by conducting a test called "optical coherence tomography" (OCT). This painless test uses light waves to take detailed pictures of your retina. Before the test, your doctor may give you some eye drops to dilate (widen) your pupil.

WHAT IS THE TREATMENT FOR A MACULAR HOLE?

If a macular hole is affecting your vision, you will likely need a type of surgery called "vitrectomy" to repair the hole and prevent permanent vision loss. Treatment works best when doctors catch macular holes early, so it is important to talk to your eye doctor right away if you notice symptoms of one.[1]

Section 13.3 | Macular Pucker

WHAT IS A MACULAR PUCKER?

A macular pucker is a rare eye condition that can cause wavy or distorted vision. Experts do not always know what causes it.

Many people with macular puckers experience mild symptoms, and most do not need treatment. However, if the pucker makes it hard to perform daily activities, surgery may help you see more clearly.

WHAT CAUSES A MACULAR PUCKER?

Most of the time, a macular pucker occurs due to normal changes in your eye as you age.

As you age, your vitreous—the clear gel that fills your eye and gives it a round shape—shrinks and pulls away from your retina (the light-sensitive layer of tissue at the back of the eye). This process is called a "vitreous detachment," and it happens to everyone as they get older.

In some people, a membrane forms on the surface of the retina. This membrane can create wrinkles or "puckers." If the membrane forms over a part of the retina called the "macula," it can cause a macular pucker.

WHAT ARE THE SYMPTOMS OF A MACULAR PUCKER?

A macular pucker can cause things to appear wavy or distorted. Straight lines—such as a sentence in a book—might look bent or wavy. When reading, you might notice that letters or words are hard to read, missing, or crowded. You may also have trouble seeing small details.

---

[1] "Macular Hole," National Eye Institute (NEI), November 15, 2023. Available online. URL: www.nei.nih.gov/learn-about-eye-health/eye-conditions-and-diseases/macular-hole. Accessed August 3, 2024.

If the macular pucker worsens, letters or objects may become so blurry that they are difficult to see.

A macular pucker usually affects one eye. In most cases, symptoms are mild and worsen slowly. Some people adjust to the changes in their vision—but if you notice any changes, it is important to talk to your eye doctor. In rare cases, a macular pucker can cause severe vision loss or lead to a related eye condition called a "macular hole."

ARE YOU AT RISK FOR A MACULAR PUCKER?

A macular pucker can occur at any age, but your risk increases as you get older.

You may also be at risk for a macular pucker if you:

- have floaters
- have had a vitreous detachment
- have had a retinal tear or retinal detachment
- have had an eye injury, laser treatment, or eye surgery
- have had uveitis (inflammation in your eye)

WHAT IS THE TREATMENT FOR A MACULAR PUCKER?

Most people with a macular pucker have mild symptoms that do not require treatment, but you must undergo regular eye exams to ensure the macular pucker does not worsen. Your eye doctor might also recommend glasses or a new glasses prescription to help you see better.

If a macular pucker significantly affects your ability to perform everyday activities, such as reading or driving, consult your eye doctor. You may need surgery to remove the membrane and smooth out the wrinkles on your retina.

There are two types of surgery for a macular pucker:

- **Vitrectomy**. During a vitrectomy, the doctor removes the vitreous and then removes the membrane from the retina.
- **Membranectomy**. During this surgery, the eye doctor removes the membrane from your retina. This procedure usually takes less than 30 minutes and can be performed in a doctor's office.[1]

---

[1] "Macular Pucker," National Eye Institute (NEI), November 15, 2023. Available online. URL: www.nei.nih.gov/learn-about-eye-health/eye-conditions-and-diseases/macular-pucker. Accessed August 3, 2024.

Chapter 14 | **Congenital Disorders and Syndromes**

Chapter Contents

Section 14.1 | Congenital Rubella

INTRODUCTION TO CONGENITAL RUBELLA

Congenital rubella refers to the group of birth defects that occur in an infant whose mother is infected with the virus that causes German measles (rubella) during pregnancy. This condition occurs when the rubella virus in the mother affects the developing baby during the first three months of pregnancy. After the fourth month, if the mother contracts a rubella infection, it is less likely to harm the developing baby.

The most common problems associated with congenital rubella include:

- hearing loss due to damage to the nerve pathways from the inner ear to the brain (sensorineural hearing loss)
- ocular abnormalities:
    - cataracts
    - infantile glaucoma
    - pigmentary retinopathy
- heart problems

Other symptoms and signs may include:

- intrauterine growth retardation
- prematurity
- stillbirth
- miscarriage
- neurological problems:
    - intellectual disability
    - low muscle tone
    - a very small head
- liver and spleen enlargement (hepatosplenomegaly)
- jaundice
- skin problems
- anemia
- hormonal problems

The number of babies born with congenital rubella has significantly decreased since the rubella vaccine was developed. However, pregnant women who are not vaccinated for rubella and who have not had the disease in the past risk infecting themselves and their unborn babies.

CAUSES OF CONGENITAL RUBELLA

Infection during Pregnancy or Childbirth

This disease is caused by an infection being passed from a pregnant person to their unborn fetus during pregnancy or to their newborn infant during childbirth. This is known as "congenital infection." Often, when a pregnant person becomes infected by a harmful virus, bacteria, fungus, or parasite, their immune system protects their fetus from the infection. However, in the case of this disease, the infection may be transmitted through the placenta or birth canal and affect the fetus/baby.

Congenital infection may be difficult to diagnose, as the pregnant person and their fetus/baby may not immediately show any symptoms. However, testing for this disease is available to the mother during pregnancy and to the baby after birth. Healthcare providers often recommend all pregnant individuals and babies get tested for this disease, even if there are no suspected symptoms.

Genetic Mutations

Congenital rubella syndrome can be caused by genetic mutations, also known as "pathogenic variants." Genetic mutations can be hereditary, passed down from parents to their children, or they may occur randomly during cell division. Genetic mutations may also result from contracted viruses, environmental factors, such as UV radiation from sunlight exposure, or a combination of these.

If you suspect you may have this disease, consider collecting your family health history. Information such as other family members who have had similar symptoms, the onset of their/your symptoms, or exposures to any potential disease-causing environmental factors should be discussed with your medical team.

SYMPTOMS OF CONGENITAL RUBELLA

The types of symptoms experienced, and their intensity may vary among individuals with this disease. Your experience may differ from others. Consult your health-care team for more information.[1]

Section 14.2 | Microcephaly

WHAT IS MICROCEPHALY?

Microcephaly is a condition where a baby's head is much smaller than expected. During pregnancy, a baby's head grows as the baby's brain grows. Microcephaly can occur because a baby's brain has not developed properly during pregnancy or stopped growing after birth. Microcephaly can occur alone or in combination with other major birth defects. The severity of microcephaly can range from mild to severe (see Figure 14.1).

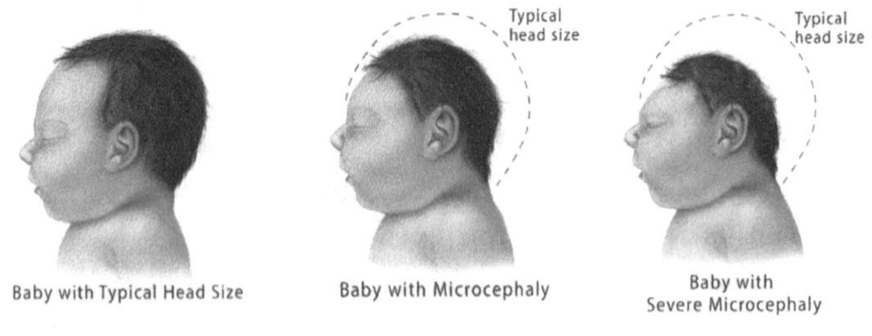

Figure 14.1. Severity of Microcephaly

Centers for Disease Control and Prevention (CDC)

[1] Genetic and Rare Diseases Information Center (GARD), "Congenital Rubella Syndrome," National Center for Advancing Translational Sciences (NCATS), July 2024. Available online. URL: https://rarediseases.info.nih.gov/diseases/4744/congenital-rubella. Accessed August 5, 2024.

SEVERE MICROCEPHALY

Severe microcephaly is a serious, extreme form of this condition and can be life-threatening.

ASSOCIATED PROBLEMS

Babies with microcephaly can have multiple health problems, depending on the severity of the condition. Some common problems include:

- seizures
- developmental delays, such as problems with speech and walking
- intellectual disability
- problems with movement and balance
- feeding problems, such as difficulty swallowing
- hearing loss
- vision problems

CAUSES OF MICROCEPHALY

The causes of microcephaly in most babies are unknown. Some known causes of microcephaly include:

- infections during pregnancy, such as Zika, toxoplasmosis, or cytomegalovirus
- malnutrition during pregnancy
- malnutrition in the baby after birth
- exposure to harmful substances, such as alcohol or certain drugs
- problems with blood supply to the baby's brain during development

DIAGNOSIS OF MICROCEPHALY

Microcephaly can be diagnosed during pregnancy through ultrasound or after the baby is born.

During Pregnancy

Prenatal diagnosis of microcephaly can be done late in the second or early in the third trimester.

After the Baby Is Born

To diagnose microcephaly after birth, a health-care provider will measure the baby's head circumference, which measures the distance around the baby's head. The provider then compares this measurement to population standards using Centers for Disease Control and Prevention's (CDC) charts (based on age and sex) or INTERGROWTH 21st (based on age, sex, and pregnancy duration). Microcephaly is defined as a head circumference that is significantly smaller than the average for babies of the same age and sex.

Commonly used birth head circumference reference charts are based on measurements taken before 24 hours of age, so it is common to measure a baby's head circumference in the first 24 hours.

Head circumference measurements may be influenced by factors related to delivery that might alter the shape of the baby's head. If the delivery affected the baby's head, a provider might wait longer than 24 hours. Widely accepted head circumference charts include the World Health Organization's (WHO) charts for children aged zero to two years.

If the health-care provider suspects microcephaly, they can request tests to help confirm the diagnosis and look for other problems. For example, magnetic resonance imaging can provide information on the structure of the baby's brain.

TREATMENT OF MICROCEPHALY

Microcephaly is a lifelong condition. There is no known cure or standard treatment. The severity of microcephaly can vary, and so can the treatment options. Babies with mild microcephaly often do not experience additional problems and will need regular checkups to monitor their growth and development.

For more severe cases, babies will need ongoing care and treatment focused on managing their health problems. Developmental services early in life often help babies with microcephaly to improve and maximize their physical and intellectual abilities. These services, known as "early intervention," can include speech, occupational, and physical therapies. Sometimes, medications are also needed to treat seizures or other symptoms.[1]

Section 14.3 | Leber Congenital Amaurosis

OVERVIEW OF LEBER CONGENITAL AMAUROSIS

Leber congenital amaurosis (LCA) is an eye disorder present from birth (congenital). This condition primarily affects the retina, the specialized tissue at the back of the eye that detects light and color. Individuals with this disorder typically experience severe visual impairment beginning at birth or shortly thereafter. The visual impairment tends to be severe and may worsen over time.

Leber congenital amaurosis is also associated with other vision problems, including:

- increased sensitivity to light (photophobia)
- involuntary movements of the eyes (nystagmus)
- extreme farsightedness (hyperopia)

Additionally, the pupils, which usually expand and contract in response to light, do not react normally. They may expand and contract more slowly than usual or may not respond to light at all.

A specific behavior called "Franceschetti's oculo-digital sign" is characteristic of LCA. This behavior involves affected individuals poking, pressing, and rubbing their eyes with a knuckle or finger, often resulting in the sensation of flashes of light called "phosphenes." Researchers suspect that this behavior may contribute to deep-set eyes in affected children.

In very rare cases, delayed development and intellectual disability have been reported in individuals with the features of LCA. Due to visual loss, affected children may become isolated. Providing opportunities for play, sensory experiences, and early educational

[1] "Microcephaly," Centers for Disease Control and Prevention (CDC), May 16, 2024. Available online. URL: www.cdc.gov/birth-defects/about/microcephaly.html. Accessed August 5, 2024.

interventions can help prevent developmental delays in children with LCA.

At least 20 genetic types of LCA have been described, distinguished by their genetic causes, patterns of vision loss, and related eye abnormalities.

CAUSES OF LEBER CONGENITAL AMAUROSIS

Leber congenital amaurosis can result from variants (also known as "mutations") in at least 20 genes, all necessary for the function of the retina and normal vision. These genes play various roles in the development and function of the retina. For example, some genes associated with this disorder are crucial for the normal development of light-detecting cells called "photoreceptors." Other genes are involved in phototransduction, the process by which light entering the eye is converted into electrical signals transmitted to the brain. Additional genes play a role in the function of cilia, which are microscopic finger-like projections that stick out from the surface of many types of cells. Cilia are found in the retina's photoreceptors and are essential for vision.

Variants in any of the genes associated with LCA disrupt the development and function of the retina, resulting in early vision loss. Variants in the *CEP290*, *CRB1*, *GUCY2D*, and *RPE65* genes are the most common causes of LCA, while variants in other genes account for a smaller percentage of cases. In about 30 percent of all people with LCA, the cause of the disorder is unknown, though research is ongoing.

FREQUENCY OF LEBER CONGENITAL AMAUROSIS

Leber congenital amaurosis occurs in two to three per 100,000 newborns. It is one of the most common causes of blindness in children.

INHERITANCE OF LEBER CONGENITAL AMAUROSIS

Leber congenital amaurosis usually follows an autosomal recessive inheritance pattern. Autosomal recessive inheritance means both copies of the gene in each cell have variants. The parents of an individual with an autosomal recessive condition each carry only one copy of the altered gene and, therefore, typically do not show any signs and symptoms of the disease.

When LCA is caused by variants in the *CRX* or *IMPDH1* genes, the disorder follows an autosomal dominant inheritance pattern. Autosomal dominant inheritance means one copy of the altered gene in each cell is sufficient to cause the disorder. In most cases, an affected person inherits a gene mutation from one affected parent. Other cases result from new variants and occur in individuals with no family history of the disorder.[1]

Section 14.4 | **Anophthalmia and Microphthalmia**

WHAT ARE ANOPHTHALMIA AND MICROPHTHALMIA?

Anophthalmia and microphthalmia are eye conditions present from birth. Anophthalmia is when a baby is born without one or both of their eyes. Microphthalmia is when one or both of a baby's eyes are abnormally small. Both conditions are rare and can cause vision loss or blindness. No treatment can create a new eye or restore vision for people born with anophthalmia or microphthalmia. However, early treatment can help babies and children with these conditions grow and develop.

CAUSES OF ANOPHTHALMIA AND MICROPHTHALMIA

Most of the time, doctors do not know what causes anophthalmia or microphthalmia. These conditions may be caused by the following:

- **Changes in genes**. Some babies have anophthalmia or microphthalmia due to genetic mutations. These changes occur during pregnancy, before the baby is born, and may also cause other birth defects.
- **Taking certain medicines during pregnancy**. Some medications can cause anophthalmia and microphthalmia if taken during pregnancy. This includes isotretinoin (Accutane, a medicine that treats severe acne) and

[1] MedlinePlus, "Leber Congenital Amaurosis," National Institutes of Health (NIH), October 6, 2022. Available online. URL: https://medlineplus.gov/genetics/condition/leber-congenital-amaurosis/#synonyms. Accessed August 5, 2024.

thalidomide (a medicine that treats certain skin problems and some types of cancer).
- Exposure to harmful environmental factors, such as:
    - x-rays
    - chemicals
    - drugs
    - pesticides
    - radiation
    - viruses

Experts believe a combination of genetic factors and environmental exposures could also cause anophthalmia and microphthalmia.

HEALTH PROBLEMS ASSOCIATED WITH ANOPHTHALMIA AND MICROPHTHALMIA

Anophthalmia and microphthalmia can cause vision problems and blindness. Individuals with these conditions may also have small eye sockets, affecting the shape of their faces. People with microphthalmia may have additional eye conditions, including:

- coloboma (missing tissue in or around the eye)
- cataract (a cloudy area in the lens of the eye)
- microcornea (a small and unusually curved clear outer layer at the front of the eye)

Individuals with anophthalmia or microphthalmia may also have birth defects that lead to other health problems.

REDUCING THE RISK OF ANOPHTHALMIA AND MICROPHTHALMIA

To reduce the risk of anophthalmia and microphthalmia, consider the following:

- getting a checkup before pregnancy
- discussing medications with your doctor
- visiting a genetic counselor to understand your genetic risks
- regular prenatal care during pregnancy
- avoiding harmful environmental exposures

DIAGNOSING ANOPHTHALMIA AND MICROPHTHALMIA

These conditions can be diagnosed either during pregnancy or shortly after birth.

During Pregnancy

Doctors can check for anophthalmia and microphthalmia using:

- ultrasound (to visualize structures in the body)
- computed tomography (CT) scan (a type of x-ray)
- genetic testing (tests on blood and other tissues to detect genetic disorders)

After the Baby Is Born

After birth, a doctor can diagnose anophthalmia or microphthalmia through a physical exam.

TREATMENT FOR ANOPHTHALMIA AND MICROPHTHALMIA

There is no treatment to create a new eye or restore vision. However, early treatment can help manage the condition.

- **Devices**. Babies and children may need special devices called "conformers" to help their eye sockets grow and develop. They may also wear a prosthetic eye for cosmetic reasons and to aid eye socket growth.
- **Protective eyewear**. For babies born with vision in only one eye, prescription eyeglasses or safety goggles are necessary to protect the functioning eye.
- **Patch**. Children with microphthalmia who retain some vision in the smaller eye may benefit from wearing a patch on the other eye to strengthen vision.
- **Surgery**. Surgical procedures may be needed to enlarge the eye socket, accommodate devices, or address other eye issues such as cataracts.[1]

[1] "Anophthalmia and Microphthalmia," National Eye Institute (NEI), November 15, 2023. Available online. URL: www.nei.nih.gov/learn-about-eye-health/eye-conditions-and-diseases/anophthalmia-and-microphthalmia. Accessed August 5, 2024.

Section 14.5 | Ocular Albinism

WHAT IS OCULAR ALBINISM?

Ocular albinism is a genetic condition that primarily affects the eyes. It reduces the pigmentation of the iris (the colored part of the eye) and the retina (the light-sensitive tissue at the back of the eye), which is essential for normal vision.

Ocular albinism is characterized by severely impaired sharpness of vision (visual acuity) and problems with combining vision from both eyes to perceive depth (stereoscopic vision). Although the vision loss is permanent, it does not worsen over time.

Other eye abnormalities associated with this condition include:

- rapid, involuntary eye movements (nystagmus)
- eyes that do not look in the same direction (strabismus)
- increased sensitivity to light (photophobia).

Many affected individuals also have abnormalities involving the optic nerves, which carry visual information from the eye to the brain.

Unlike some other forms of albinism, ocular albinism does not significantly affect the color of the skin and hair. People with this condition may have a somewhat lighter complexion than other members of their family, but these differences are usually minor.

The most common form of ocular albinism is known as the "Nettleship-Falls type" or "type 1." Other forms are much rarer and may be associated with additional signs and symptoms, such as hearing loss.

CAUSES OF OCULAR ALBINISM

Ocular albinism type 1 results from mutations in the *GPR143* gene. This gene provides instructions for making a protein involved in the pigmentation of the eyes and skin. It helps control the growth of melanosomes, which are cellular structures that produce and store a pigment called "melanin." Melanin gives skin, hair, and eyes their color. In the retina, this pigment also plays a role in normal vision.

Most mutations in the *GPR143* gene alter the size or shape of the *GPR143* protein. Many of these genetic changes prevent the protein from reaching melanosomes to control their growth. In other cases, the protein reaches melanosomes normally, but mutations disrupt the protein's function. As a result of these changes, melanosomes in skin cells and the retina can grow abnormally large. Researchers are uncertain how these giant melanosomes are related to vision loss and other eye abnormalities in people with ocular albinism.

Rare cases of ocular albinism are not caused by mutations in the *GPR143* gene. In these cases, the genetic cause of the condition is often unknown.

FREQUENCY OF OCULAR ALBINISM

The most common form of this disorder, ocular albinism type 1, affects at least 1 in 60,000 males. The classic signs and symptoms of this condition are much less common in females.

INHERITANCE OF OCULAR ALBINISM

Ocular albinism type 1 is inherited in an X-linked pattern. A condition is considered X-linked if the mutated gene that causes the disorder is located on the X chromosome, one of the two sex chromosomes. In males (who have only one X chromosome), one altered copy of the *GPR143* gene in each cell is sufficient to cause the characteristic features of ocular albinism. Because females have two copies of the X chromosome, women with only one copy of a *GPR143* mutation in each cell usually do not experience vision loss or other significant eye abnormalities. They may have mild changes in retinal pigmentation that can be detected during an eye examination.[1]

[1] MedlinePlus, "Ocular Albinism," National Institutes of Health (NIH), November 1, 2017. Available online. URL: https://medlineplus.gov/genetics/condition/ocular-albinism. Accessed August 5, 2024.

Chapter 15 | Strabismus (Crossed Eyes)

Crossed eyes, or strabismus, is a disorder in which the eyes are misaligned and point in different directions. One eye may point in a straight direction, while the other points inward, outward, upward, or downward direction. The eye that points straight and the misaligned one can differ. Strabismus is common among children, with about 4 percent of children in the United States affected by this disorder.

TYPES OF STRABISMUS

The types of strabismus are as follows.

Esotropia

Esotropia is further classified into infantile esotropia and accommodative esotropia. Infantile esotropia occurs when the eyes turn inward, a common type of strabismus in infants. Accommodative esotropia is a common form of strabismus that occurs in children two years of age or older. In this case, the eye turns inward when the child tries to focus on something, either at a distance or up close.

Exotropia

Exotropia is a condition in which the eye turns outward, often occurring when a child focuses on distant objects. This usually happens when a child is daydreaming, ill, or tired. The child may also squint one eye to see more clearly in bright sunlight.

CAUSES OF STRABISMUS

Strabismus is commonly attributed to issues with the brain's control of eye movement or eye muscle–related issues. The condition is common in children with Down syndrome, cerebral palsy (CP), brain tumor, and hydrocephalus. A few other causes of strabismus are as follows:

- **Heredity**. A family history of strabismus or other similar ocular diseases can increase the likelihood of developing strabismus. Genetic factors may influence abnormalities in eye muscle control or visual development.
- **Refractive error**. Individuals with farsightedness strain their eyes to focus clearly, which can lead to the development of strabismus.
- **Weakness of muscles.** Muscular dysfunction or weakness affecting the regulation of eye movement can either be present from birth or develop later in life as a result of trauma, nerve impairment, or neurological disorders.
- **Injuries**. Eye injuries or procedures involving the eye or orbit can cause a disturbance in the normal functioning of the eye muscles and nerves, resulting in strabismus.

SYMPTOMS OF STRABISMUS

The main symptom of strabismus is that the eyes do not aim in the same direction, causing squinting in one eye in bright sunlight, or tilting the head to use the eyes together. Other symptoms include:

- double vision
- uncoordinated movement of the eyes
- loss of vision or perception of depth

If any of these symptoms are noticed, immediate help from an eye doctor should be sought.

DIAGNOSIS OF STRABISMUS

Strabismus diagnosis usually entails a thorough eye examination conducted by an ophthalmologist or optometrist.

- **History of patients.** The doctor examines the patient's medical records, which includes any past eye conditions, as well as their overall health condition.

- **Visual acuity**. This involves evaluating the visual acuity of each eye by employing a standardized eye chart. Visual acuity testing is used to identify any refractive problems.
- **Conduction of cover test**. During a cover test, the physician will sequentially cover one eye at a time and carefully monitor the movement of the uncovered eye. This test aids in identifying any misalignment or deviation of the eye while the eyes are not focused on an object.
- **Evaluation of ocular alignment**. Several techniques can be used to evaluate eye alignment, including using light sources or specialized tools. These tests assist in determining the direction and magnitude of misalignment in the eyes.

It is important to note that if there is a family history of vision problems, the child needs to be examined even earlier.

TREATMENT FOR STRABISMUS

Treatment for strabismus depends on several factors, including the severity of the misalignment, the underlying cause, and the individual's age. Following are some common treatment options:

- **Eyeglasses or contact lenses**. The first step in treating those affected with strabismus is prescribing glasses to them if required. For some, this may be the only treatment required for a permanent cure.
- **Prism lenses**. These can be added to glasses to help redirect light and alleviate double vision caused by strabismus. They can also help compensate for minor misalignments.
- **Eye patches**. If strabismus is associated with amblyopia, covering the stronger eye with a patch can help strengthen the weaker eye.
- **Surgery**. Strabismus surgery involves adjusting the position of the eye muscles to realign the eyes. This surgery is used for individuals with persistent or severe

misalignment that cannot be corrected with other treatments.
- **Vision therapy**. Eye exercises and vision training techniques can help improve eye coordination and strengthen eye muscles, which may reduce the effects of strabismus.

It is important to remember that strabismus does not disappear with time and may worsen if not treated. Early treatment should be sought if any of these symptoms are present to protect vision and prevent further issues.

References

Lusby, Franklin W. "Strabismus," MedlinePlus, August 22, 2022. Available online. URL: https://medlineplus.gov/ency/article/001004.htm. Accessed August 7, 2024.

Puente, Michael A. "What Is Adult Strabismus?" American Academy of Ophthalmology (AAO), November 13, 2023. Available online. URL: www.aao.org/eye-health/diseases/what-is-strabismus. Accessed August 7, 2024.

"Strabismus (Crossed Eyes)," American Optometric Association (AOA), June 25, 2013. Available online. URL: www.aoa.org/patients-and-public/eye-and-vision-problems/glossary-of-eye-and-vision-conditions/strabismus. Accessed August 7, 2024.

Chapter 16 | Stroke and Vision Impairment

A stroke is a medical emergency that occurs when blood flow to the brain is compromised. While a stroke often results in motor and cognitive dysfunctions, its effect on vision is sometimes overlooked. Depending on the location and severity of the stroke, both neural and vascular pathways, which are essential for normal vision, can be affected, resulting in a range of visual impairments. It is crucial to understand the relationship between stroke and vision impairment for timely diagnosis and treatment of vision-related issues, thereby preventing further vision impairments.

TYPES OF VISION IMPAIRMENTS AFTER STROKE

The major types of vision impairments that may occur after a stroke are as follows:

- **Central vision loss.** This is the reduction or absence of vision in the central area of the visual field, while the peripheral vision remains unaffected. This might affect either one or both eyes.
- **Eye movement issues.** This occurs when the nerves and muscles responsible for controlling eye movements are injured as a result of stroke, leading to challenges in tracking a moving object, maintaining eye fixation, or experiencing double vision.
- **Visual field loss.** This can appear as partial or complete loss of vision in one or both eyes. The location of the stroke determines which part of the visual field is affected.
- **Homonymous hemianopia.** This is the loss of vision on the same side of the visual field in both eyes. If the stroke

affects the right side of the brain, the individual might lose vision on the left side in both eyes.

- **Homonymous quadrantanopia.** In this condition, the loss of vision occurs in the same quadrant of the visual field in both eyes. If the upper right quadrant is affected, the individual will lose vision in the upper right quadrant of both eyes.
- **Scotoma.** Also known as "blind spot," this condition involves the development of blind spots in the visual field.
- **Visual neglect.** Also known as "hemispatial neglect," this condition involves a lack of awareness of one side of an individual's own body, usually the side opposite to the brain injury. This can result in the individual not recognizing objects or people on that side, leading to difficulties with daily activities.
- **Visual agnosia.** This is a condition where the individual has difficulty recognizing or identifying familiar objects or people due to strokes affecting the visual processing areas of the brain despite having normal vision.
- **Diplopia.** Some stroke survivors may experience double vision due to damage to nerves controlling eye movement.
- **Blurred vision.** Stroke-related damage to the visual processing areas of the brain can cause blurred or distorted vision.

TREATMENT AND REHABILITATION

The treatment options for vision impairment after a stroke usually depend on the specific type and severity of the visual challenges. Some of the common treatments and rehabilitation include:

- **Prism lenses.** These lenses can be prescribed to help individuals with visual field loss or double vision. By altering the path of light entering the eyes, prism lenses can shift the visual field or align images to reduce double vision. Optometrists or ophthalmologists can determine the appropriate prism prescription based on the individual's specific visual needs.

- **Visual rehabilitation therapy (VRT)**. This therapy involves exercises and activities specifically designed to enhance visual processing, eye movement coordination, and overall visual function to promote adaptation to visual impairments caused by a stroke.
- **Medication and surgery**. Medications or surgical interventions may be necessary to address specific vision-related complications of stroke, such as increased intraocular pressure or ocular misalignment.
- **Occupational therapy**. This therapy can help stroke survivors change their daily activities to accommodate visual impairments. This may involve modifying the home environment, teaching techniques for organizing tasks, and providing training in adaptive technology.

Understanding the various effects of stroke on vision is crucial. Treatments such as lenses and therapy can enhance the quality of life (QOL) for stroke survivors dealing with vision issues. Being aware of these challenges enables individuals to seek appropriate aid promptly, leading to improved overall well-being.

References

Johnson, Jon. "What to Know about Vision Problems after Stroke," Medical News Today, January 26, 2022. Available online. URL: www.medicalnewstoday.com/articles/vision-problems-after-stroke. Accessed August 7, 2024.

Marcin, Ashley. "Vision Loss after Stroke: Why It Happens and How to Cope with It," Healthline, December 2, 2022. Available online. URL: www.healthline.com/health/vision-loss-after-stroke. Accessed August 7, 2024.

Moawad, Heidi. "Vision Changes Caused by Stroke," Verywell Health, July 25, 2023. Available online. URL: www.verywellhealth.com/vision-changes-after-stroke-4084889. Accessed August 7, 2024.

"Stroke," National Institute of Neurological Disorders and Stroke (NINDS), November 28, 2023. Available online. URL: www.ninds.nih.gov/health-information/disorders/stroke. Accessed August 7, 2024.

Part 3 | Treatment and Rehabilitation for Vision Impairment

Chapter 17 | Vision Loss Assessment

THE IMPORTANCE OF ACCURATE DIAGNOSIS IN VISION REHABILITATION

Accurate diagnosis facilitates the prescription of services, as it can illuminate factors underlying visual impairment. Understanding the cognitive, motor, and sensory interactions between vision and functioning can help target appropriate rehabilitation services. Moreover, diagnosis is tied to access to services since the allocation of public benefits and health services planning is typically based on clinical measurement.

DIAGNOSTIC RECOMMENDATIONS AND EVIDENCE

There are various authoritative recommendations regarding the diagnosis and screening of vision impairment, such as including visual assessments in general evaluations (particularly among the elderly) and training general assessors in vision rehabilitation availability. However, these are not uniformly based on strong evidence. For example, in a randomized controlled trial (RCT) of office-based screening for common problems in older persons, family physicians and internists provided with specific screening information were less likely to detect visual impairment than those in a control group. They were, however, more likely to detect hearing impairments. This discrepancy may have been due to the lower sensitivity of the screening tool used in the RCT (the MOS SF-36) for vision impairments compared to hearing impairments.

INTERVENTIONS AND COMPARATIVE STUDIES

In an unpublished study, Amy Horowitz, DSW, Senior Vice President for Research, and Director, Arlene R. Gordon Research Institute, Lighthouse International, and coworker reported on a quasi-experimental design where one nursing home served as the intervention site, receiving a three-pronged intervention, and another served as a comparison site. The intervention included:

- staff training to identify visual problems in residents
- provision of standard eye care services to avoid "excess" disability due to simple refraction error
- provision of low-vision clinical and rehabilitation teaching services to minimize the functional implications of vision loss

The staff training did not significantly improve the identification of visual problems. The intervention site, which relied on an optometrist aware of the project goals, recommended more residents for new refraction than the comparison site, which had an ophthalmologist focused on medical eye disorders. The optometrist was also more inclusive in referring visually impaired residents for rehabilitation services, unlike the ophthalmologist who reserved referrals for those more severely impaired. While there were selective improvements in patients referred for low vision clinical and rehabilitation services, comparisons of the effect of these interventions were flawed due to the referral process.

THE ROLE OF ECOLOGICAL EVALUATIONS

Ecological evaluations, where rehabilitation professionals observe clients in their surroundings, are recommended. However, the effectiveness of this assessment method remains to be substantiated with evidence.

ENTRY POINTS AND CHALLENGES IN VISION REHABILITATION

Entry into the system for vision rehabilitation often occurs through referrals from ophthalmologists, optometrists, or outreach in schools for children. The literature emphasizes the need for providers outside the vision specialties, particularly geriatricians and nursing home staff, to recognize and address vision loss. However, identifying individuals needing vision rehabilitation services remains a significant challenge. This challenge is partly due to the need for further development, validation, and recognition of instruments to assess vision impairment and related functional status. Although a few validated instruments exist for assessing functioning and satisfaction, a definitive set is not widely used.

ASSESSMENT TOOLS AND THEIR LIMITATIONS

Several tools are used to assess vision impairment and its effect, including:

- **Functional Vision Screening Questionnaire**. A brief, validated instrument focusing on functional indicators of vision problems.
- **Visual function index (VF-14)**. Measures functional impairment caused by cataracts and has shown reliability and validity.
- **NEI-VFQ**. Used to measure functional status and quality of life (QOL) in various chronic eye diseases.
- **Low Vision Functional Status Evaluation (LVSFE)**. Includes everyday tasks but needs further development for reliability and validity.
- **Low Vision Quality of Life Questionnaire (LVQOL)**. A vision-specific QOL tool with high internal consistency and good reliability.

The need for accurate screening and diagnosis poses a challenge to delivering rehabilitation services and eligibility for public benefits. This challenge extends beyond measuring vision loss to include a lack of awareness or reluctance among those at risk for low vision to be screened or diagnosed.[1]

[1] Agency for Healthcare Research and Quality (AHRQ), "Vision Rehabilitation: Care and Benefit Plan Models: Literature Review," U.S. Department of Health and Human Services (HHS), September 2012. Available online. URL: www.ahrq.gov/prevention/resources/vision/resources/vision2.html. Accessed August 6, 2024.

Chapter 18 | Managing Diabetes to Prevent Vision Loss

WHAT IS DIABETIC EYE DISEASE?

Diabetic eye disease is a group of eye problems that can affect people with diabetes. These conditions include diabetic retinopathy (DR), diabetic macular edema (DME), cataracts, and glaucoma. Over time, diabetes can cause damage to your eyes that can lead to poor vision or even blindness. However, you can take steps to prevent diabetic eye disease or keep it from getting worse by managing your diabetes.

The best ways to manage your diabetes and keep your eyes healthy are to:

- manage your blood glucose, blood pressure, and cholesterol, sometimes called the "diabetes ABCs"
- quit smoking if you smoke
- have a dilated eye exam once a year

Often, when damage first develops, there are no warning signs of diabetic eye disease or vision loss. A full, dilated eye exam helps your doctor find and treat eye problems early—often before significant vision loss can occur.

HOW DOES DIABETES AFFECT YOUR EYES?

Diabetes affects your eyes when your blood glucose, also called "blood sugar," is too high.

In the short term, vision loss from high blood glucose is not likely. However, people sometimes have blurry vision for a few days or weeks when they change their diabetes care plan or medicines. High glucose can change fluid levels or cause swelling in the tissues of your eyes that help you focus, causing blurred vision. This type of blurry vision is temporary and goes away when your glucose level gets closer to normal.

If your blood glucose stays high over time, it can damage the tiny blood vessels in the back of your eyes. This damage can begin during prediabetes when blood glucose is higher than normal but not high enough for you to be diagnosed with diabetes. Damaged blood vessels may leak fluid and cause swelling. New, weak blood vessels may also begin to grow. These blood vessels can bleed into the middle part of the eye, lead to scarring, or cause dangerously high pressure inside your eye.

Most serious diabetic eye diseases begin with blood vessel problems. The four eye diseases that can threaten your sight are:

Diabetic Retinopathy

The retina is the inner lining at the back of each eye. It senses light and turns it into signals that your brain decodes so you can see the world around you. Damaged blood vessels can harm the retina, causing a disease called "diabetic retinopathy."

In early DR, blood vessels can weaken, bulge, or leak into the retina. This stage is called "nonproliferative diabetic retinopathy."

If the disease gets worse, some blood vessels close off, which causes new blood vessels to grow or proliferate on the surface of the retina. This stage is called "proliferative diabetic retinopathy." These abnormal new blood vessels can lead to serious vision problems.

Diabetic Macular Edema

The part of your retina that you need for reading, driving, and seeing faces is called the "macula." Diabetes can lead to swelling in the macula, called "diabetic macular edema." Over time, this disease can destroy the sharp vision in this part of the eye, leading to partial vision loss or blindness. Macular edema usually develops in people who already have other signs of DR.

Glaucoma

Glaucoma is a group of eye diseases that can damage the optic nerve—the bundle of nerves that connects the eye to the brain.

Diabetes doubles the chances of having glaucoma, which can lead to vision loss and blindness if not treated early.

Cataracts

The lenses within our eyes are clear structures that help provide sharp vision, but they tend to become cloudy as we age. People with diabetes are more likely to develop cloudy lenses, called "cataracts," and they can develop cataracts at an earlier age than people without diabetes. Researchers think that high glucose levels cause deposits to build up in the lenses of your eyes.

HOW COMMON IS DIABETIC EYE DISEASE?

Diabetic Retinopathy

About one in three people with diabetes older than age 40 already have some signs of DR. DR is the most common cause of vision loss in people with diabetes. Finding and treating DR early can reduce the risk of blindness by 95 percent.

Glaucoma and Cataracts

Your chances of developing glaucoma or cataracts are about twice that of someone without diabetes.

WHO IS MORE LIKELY TO DEVELOP DIABETIC EYE DISEASE?

Anyone with diabetes can develop diabetic eye disease. Your risk is greater with:

- high blood glucose that is not treated
- high blood pressure (HBP) that is not treated

High blood cholesterol and smoking may also raise your risk for diabetic eye disease.

Some groups are affected more than others. African Americans, American Indians and Alaska Natives, Hispanics/Latinos, Pacific Islanders, and older adults are at greater risk of losing vision or going blind from diabetes.

If you have diabetes and become pregnant, you can develop eye problems very quickly. If you already have some DR, it can get worse during pregnancy. Changes that help your body support a growing baby may put stress on the blood vessels in your eyes. Your health-care team will suggest regular eye exams during pregnancy to catch and treat problems early and protect your vision.

Diabetes that occurs only during pregnancy, called "gestational diabetes," does not usually cause eye problems. Researchers are not sure why this is the case.

Your chances of developing diabetic eye disease increase the longer you have diabetes.

WHAT ARE THE SYMPTOMS OF DIABETIC EYE DISEASE?

Often, there are no early symptoms of diabetic eye disease. You may have no pain and no change in your vision as damage begins to grow inside your eyes, particularly with DR.

When symptoms do occur, they may include:

- blurry or wavy vision
- frequently changing vision—sometimes from day to day
- dark areas or vision loss
- poor color vision
- spots or dark strings (also called "floaters")
- flashes of light

Talk with your eye doctor if you have any of these symptoms.

WHEN SHOULD YOU SEE A DOCTOR RIGHT AWAY?

Call a doctor immediately if you notice sudden changes to your vision, including light flashes or many more spots (floaters) than usual. You also should see a doctor right away if it looks like a curtain is pulled over your eyes. These changes in your sight can be symptoms of a detached retina, which is a medical emergency.

HOW DO DOCTORS DIAGNOSE EYE PROBLEMS FROM DIABETES?

Having a full, dilated eye exam is the best way to check for eye problems from diabetes. Your doctor will place drops in your eyes to widen your pupils. This allows the doctor to examine a larger area at the back of each eye using a special magnifying lens. Your vision will be blurry for a few hours after a dilated exam.

Your doctor will also:

- test your vision
- measure the pressure in your eyes

HOW DO DOCTORS TREAT DIABETIC EYE DISEASE?

Your doctor may recommend having eye exams more often than once a year, along with managing your diabetes. This means managing your diabetes ABCs, which include your A1c, blood pressure, and cholesterol, and quitting smoking. Ask your health-care team what you can do to reach your goals.

Doctors may treat advanced eye problems with medicine, laser treatments, surgery, or a combination of these options.

WHAT CAN YOU DO TO PROTECT YOUR EYES?

To prevent diabetic eye disease or to keep it from getting worse, manage your diabetes ABCs: your A1c, blood pressure, and cholesterol; and quit smoking if you smoke.

Also, have a dilated eye exam at least once a year—or more often if recommended by your eye care professional. These actions are powerful ways to protect the health of your eyes and prevent blindness.

The sooner you work to manage your diabetes and other health conditions, the better. Even if you have struggled in the past to manage your health, taking better care of yourself now can protect your eyes for the future. It is never too late to begin.[1]

[1] "Diabetic Eye Disease," National Institute of Diabetes and Digestive and Kidney Diseases (NIDDK), May 2017. Available online. URL: www.niddk.nih.gov/health-information/diabetes/overview/preventing-problems/diabetic-eye-disease#treat. Accessed August 6, 2024.

Chapter 19 | **Surgical Interventions**

Chapter Contents

Section 19.1 | Cataract Surgery

A cataract is a cloudy area in the lens of your eye—the clear part of the eye that helps to focus light. This can make your vision appear cloudy. Surgery is the only way to remove cataracts.

WHO NEEDS CATARACT SURGERY?

Your eye doctor will probably suggest cataract surgery if you experience vision loss that interferes with everyday activities such as reading, driving, or watching TV.

Your doctor might also recommend surgery even if your cataracts are not the primary cause of your vision problems. For example, you may need to remove cataracts, so your doctor can examine the back of your eye. This examination can help them monitor and treat other eye conditions, such as diabetic retinopathy (DR) or age-related macular degeneration (AMD).

There is no need to rush into surgery to remove cataracts. Ask your eye doctor about the risks and benefits of cataract surgery to decide if it is right for you.

Keep in mind that if you have cataracts in both eyes, you will need to undergo surgery on each eye at separate times, usually about a month apart.

HOW DO YOU PREPARE FOR CATARACT SURGERY?

You will likely need to take several steps to prepare for your cataract surgery. Your eye doctor will provide specific instructions.

Before Your Surgery

- **Visit your eye doctor**. About a week before your surgery, your eye doctor will perform tests to measure the size and shape of your eye. These tests help your doctor choose the appropriate type of artificial lens (called an "intraocular lens" or "IOL").
- **Use special eye drops**. Your eye doctor may prescribe these drops to help prevent infections.

- **Stop taking certain medications.** Inform your eye doctor about any medications you are taking. If you are taking a medication that could cause bleeding during your surgery, your doctor may ask you to stop taking it temporarily.
- **Do not eat or drink the night before.** Your doctor may instruct you to stop eating and drinking several hours before your surgery.
- **Clean your eyelids and eyelashes.** The night before and the morning of your surgery, you may need to clean your eyelids and eyelashes with baby shampoo to eliminate any germs that could cause an infection.

The Day of Your Surgery

Be sure to bring a friend or family member with you on the day of your surgery. You will not be able to drive afterward, so you will need someone to ensure you get home safely.

WHAT HAPPENS DURING CATARACT SURGERY?

During surgery, your eye doctor will remove the cloudy lens from your eye and replace it with an artificial lens (an intraocular lens or IOL). The procedure lasts about one hour and is almost painless.

Typically, you will be awake during cataract surgery. You might notice lights or movement, but you will not be able to see what your doctor is doing. Your eye doctor can administer medication to help you stay relaxed and calm during the procedure.

During the surgery, your eye doctor will:

- Apply numbing drops to your eye to prevent any sensation of pain.
- Use tiny tools to make an incision in your eye, break up the lens, and remove it.
- Insert the new artificial lens into your eye.

After the lens is in place, you will rest for a short period in a recovery area outside the operating room. Before you leave, the medical team will check to ensure there are no complications with your eye.

WHAT HAPPENS AFTER CATARACT SURGERY?

Your eye doctor will explain how to care for your eye following cataract surgery. They will prescribe eye drops to aid in healing, and you may need to wear a special eye shield or glasses. You should also avoid certain activities for a few weeks—such as touching your eye, bending over, or lifting heavy objects.

Your eye may feel slightly itchy or uncomfortable and be sensitive to light and touch. Typically, these sensations improve within one or two days.

Contact your eye doctor immediately if you experience any of the following symptoms after surgery:

- vision loss
- severe pain that does not subside with medication
- extremely red eyes
- floaters—flashes of light or numerous small dark spots or squiggly lines that float across your vision

Most people fully recover eight weeks after their surgery. Your eye doctor will schedule follow-up appointments to ensure your eye is healing properly.

WILL YOUR VISION BE NORMAL AFTER CATARACT SURGERY?

Approximately 9 out of 10 people who undergo cataract surgery experience improved vision, although you may initially have blurry vision while your eye heals.

After cataract surgery, some individuals notice that colors appear brighter. This is because the artificial lens does not have the noticeable yellow or brown tint that your natural lens had due to the cataract.

Once your eye has completely healed, you might need a new prescription for glasses or contact lenses to see clearly.

WHAT ARE THE RISKS OF CATARACT SURGERY?

Cataract surgery is among the most common, safe, and effective surgeries performed in the United States. However, as with any surgery, there are risks. These can include:

- swelling, bleeding, or infections
- vision loss or double vision

- unusual changes in eye pressure
- retinal detachment
- secondary cataracts (posterior capsule opacity)

It is crucial to address these issues promptly. Be sure to attend all your scheduled checkups and contact your eye doctor if you notice any issues with your eyes or vision.[1]

Section 19.2 | Corneal Transplantation

WHAT IS A CORNEAL TRANSPLANT?

If you have severe damage to your cornea—the clear front layer of your eye—doctors can replace the damaged part with healthy corneal tissue from a donor.

If you have scarring or other damage that affects the entire cornea, doctors can perform a full-thickness corneal transplant (called a "penetrating keratoplasty"). If only part of your cornea is damaged, doctors can conduct a partial thickness transplant (called a "lamellar keratoplasty").

WHAT HAPPENS DURING A CORNEAL TRANSPLANT?

You may receive general anesthesia to put you to sleep during the transplant surgery, or you may be awake. If you are awake, your doctor will administer medication to numb your eye and another medicine to help you relax.

Your doctor will use a special tool to keep your eye open during surgery. They will remove the damaged part of your cornea and replace it with healthy donor tissue.

[1] "Cataract Surgery," National Eye Institute (NEI), January 4, 2023. Available online. URL: www.nei.nih.gov/learn-about-eye-health/eye-conditions-and-diseases/cataracts/cataract-surgery. Accessed August 5, 2024.

RECOVERY PROCESS

A corneal transplant is an outpatient surgery that allows you to go home the same day. However, you will not be able to drive, so you will need someone to transport you home after the surgery.

You will require a follow-up appointment the day after surgery to check on your eye's healing progress.

POSTOPERATIVE CARE

After surgery, it is crucial to take steps to aid your eye's recovery:

- Use special eye drops prescribed by your doctor.
- Avoid rubbing or pressing on your eye.
- Wear eyeglasses or a special shield to protect your eye.

Depending on the type of transplant, full recovery can take up to a year. Discuss with your doctor when you can resume your normal activities.

WHEN TO SEEK IMMEDIATE HELP

Corneal rejection can manifest as:

- eye pain
- sensitivity to light
- red eyes
- cloudy or hazy vision

If you experience these symptoms after a corneal transplant, inform your eye doctor immediately.

POTENTIAL SIDE EFFECTS

Like any surgery, corneal transplant surgery carries risks. One major risk is tissue rejection, where your body perceives the new cornea as a foreign object and attempts to reject it. Your doctor can prescribe medication to help prevent rejection and preserve your cornea.

Corneal transplants can also lead to other eye problems, including:

- infection
- eye bleeding
- retinal detachment
- glaucoma

If you experience tissue rejection or other severe issues with your new cornea, you may require another transplant. Discuss the risks of a corneal transplant with your doctor to determine if this treatment is appropriate for you.[1]

Section 19.3 | Glaucoma Surgery

Glaucoma is a group of eye diseases that can cause vision loss and blindness by damaging the optic nerve in the back of your eye.

If glaucoma medications and laser treatment have not been effective, your doctor may recommend surgery. While surgery cannot cure glaucoma or reverse vision loss, it can help protect your vision from further deterioration.

TYPES OF GLAUCOMA SURGERY

There are several types of surgery for glaucoma that aim to reduce eye pressure:

- trabeculectomy
- glaucoma implant surgery
- minimally invasive glaucoma surgery (MIGS)

If you require surgery in both eyes, your doctor will operate on one eye at a time.

Trabeculectomy

Trabeculectomy is commonly used to treat open-angle glaucoma. It is performed in a hospital and usually takes less than an hour.

During this procedure, the surgeon creates a small opening in the top of your eye, hidden under your eyelid to make it unnoticeable. This opening allows excess fluid to drain from your eye, reducing pressure.

---

[1] "Corneal Transplants," National Eye Institute (NEI), July 5, 2019. Available online. URL: www.nei.nih.gov/learn-about-eye-health/eye-conditions-and-diseases/corneal-conditions/corneal-transplants. Accessed August 5, 2024.

Patients are typically awake during this surgery, receiving numbing medication and sedatives. Most individuals can go home the same day but will need someone to drive them.

Glaucoma Implant Surgery

This surgery is applicable for various types of glaucoma, including congenital, neovascular, and trauma-induced glaucoma. It generally lasts between one and two hours.

A tiny tube or shunt is implanted onto the white part of your eye to help drain excess fluid, thus lowering the eye pressure.

Like trabeculectomy, patients are awake during the procedure, receive numbing medication, and can usually go home the same day, provided they have transportation.

Minimally Invasive Glaucoma Surgery

For patients with mild glaucoma, MIGS offers a lower-risk option with fewer side effects and a quicker recovery time.

There are various types of MIGS, and it is essential to discuss with your eye doctor whether this could be a viable option for you.

WHAT HAPPENS AFTER SURGERY?

Your doctor will prescribe eye drops to help prevent swelling and infections. You will need to use them for several weeks. These eye drops differ from other glaucoma eye drops you may already use.

While you recover, you may need to avoid some activities for two to four weeks, such as lifting anything heavy. You will also need check-ups with your doctor to ensure your eye is healing well.

WILL I NEED SURGERY AGAIN?

For some people, the benefits of surgery last a long time. For others, the opening in the eye begins to close up, and they need surgery again. You will need regular check-ups with your doctor to test your eye pressure. That way, your doctor can act fast if you need more treatment.

Research shows that trabeculectomy can lower eye pressure in about 7 out of 10 people. It may work best in people without an eye injury or another eye surgery.

WHAT ARE THE SIDE EFFECTS OF SURGERY FOR GLAUCOMA?

Glaucoma surgery can have side effects, just like any operation. For example, your eye may be swollen and sore for a while.

Other possible risks of glaucoma surgery include:

- cataract
- problems with the cornea (the clear front layer of your eye)
- eye pressure that is too low
- vision loss

Talk over the pros and cons of surgery with your doctor. Together, you can make a treatment plan that is right for you.[1]

Section 19.4 | LASIK (Laser-Assisted in Situ Keratomileusis)

WHAT IS LASIK?

Laser-assisted in situ keratomileusis (LASIK) uses a laser (a strong beam of light) to change the shape of the cornea and help make vision clearer. It works best for adults with nearsightedness, farsightedness, or astigmatism. It cannot fix presbyopia. For LASIK to work correctly, your vision must be stable (meaning your eyeglass or contact lens prescription stays the same over time).

IS LASIK RIGHT FOR YOU?

To find out if LASIK is right for you, you will need a comprehensive dilated eye exam. The exam is simple and painless. Your eye doctor will ask you to read letters that are up close and far away. Then they will give you some eye drops to dilate (widen) your pupil and check for other eye problems.

[1] "Glaucoma Surgery," National Eye Institute (NEI), January 3, 2022. Available online. URL: www.nei.nih.gov/learn-about-eye-health/eye-conditions-and-diseases/glaucoma/glaucoma-surgery. Accessed August 5, 2024.

Laser-assisted in situ keratomileusis is not right for everyone. Some eye conditions can raise your risk for complications from LASIK, including:

- **Keratoconus**. A disease that makes the cornea thinner over time.
- **Eye infections**. Such as keratitis or ocular herpes.
- **Dry eye**. Chronic dryness of the eyes.
- **Glaucoma**. A condition that damages the optic nerve.
- **Cataract**. Clouding of the lens in the eye.
- **Large pupils**. Can affect night vision and increase the risk of glare.

Talk with your eye doctor to decide if LASIK or another type of refractive surgery is right for you.

WHAT ARE THE BENEFITS OF LASIK?

After LASIK, most people see well enough to stop wearing eyeglasses or contact lenses for most of their daily activities. Since everyone gets presbyopia as they age, and LASIK cannot fix presbyopia, most people will still need single-vision glasses or contact lenses at some point.

WHAT ARE THE RISKS OF LASIK?

LASIK can cause side effects, just like any surgery. Common side effects include:

- **Dry eye**. A sensation of dryness in the eyes.
- **Seeing a glare or halo around bright lights**. Especially at night.
- **Double vision**. Seeing two images of a single object.
- **Blurry vision**. Temporary blurriness after surgery.
- **Sensitivity to light**. Increased discomfort from light exposure.

These side effects usually go away after a few months. Your eye doctor may give you eye drops or other medicines to help with them. Rarely, these problems can be permanent.

Other risks of LASIK include:

- **Infection.** Risk of eye infection after the surgery.
- **Problems with corneal healing.** Delayed or incomplete healing.
- **Vision loss.** Seeing less clearly than before surgery.

If LASIK causes vision loss, you may need another surgery to fix it. Rarely, vision loss from LASIK may be permanent.

If you see clearly with eyeglasses or contacts, you may decide that the risks of LASIK outweigh the benefits. Talk with your eye doctor about the risks and benefits and decide together if surgery is right for you.

WHAT HAPPENS DURING LASIK SURGERY?

During an eye exam before the surgery, your eye doctor will use a scanner to make a detailed image of your cornea. This image will guide the laser during surgery.

Just before surgery, your doctor will put drops in your eye to numb it. They may also give you medicine to help you relax.

During the surgery, your doctor will cut a small flap in your cornea and fold it back. Then, they will shine a laser into your eye, programmed to change your cornea into the correct shape. Then, they will put the corneal flap back in place.

HOW LONG DOES IT TAKE TO RECOVER?

Right after surgery, your eye might be irritated, and your vision will be blurry, so you will need someone to give you a ride home from the doctor's office.

Your eye doctor may give you medicine or special eye drops to help with any pain after the surgery. You may also need to wear a special patch over your eye for several nights to protect it while you sleep.

You will be able to see after surgery, but it takes two to three months for your eye to finish healing. Your vision will get clearer as your eye heals. Ask your doctor about when you can go back to your normal activities.

Your eye doctor can talk with you about the different types and the risks and benefits of surgery. It is important to discuss your specific eye health and vision goals with your eye doctor to determine if LASIK or another type of refractive surgery is the best choice for you.[1]

Section 19.5 | Vitrectomy

If you have an eye condition that affects your retina (the light-sensitive layer of tissue at the back of your eye) or vitreous (the gel-like fluid that fills your eye), your eye doctor may recommend a type of surgery called "vitrectomy."

WHAT EYE CONDITIONS DOES VITRECTOMY TREAT?

Vitrectomy can help doctors treat several eye conditions. For example, vitrectomy may be part of the treatment plan for:

- **Retinal detachment**. Helps your doctor repair any holes or tears in the retina.
- **Diabetic retinopathy (DR)**. Replaces cloudy vitreous and helps your doctor find and repair sources of bleeding in the retina.

Like any surgery, this treatment has risks. Talk with your doctor about the risks and benefits of vitrectomy.

WHAT HAPPENS DURING VITRECTOMY?

During vitrectomy surgery, your eye doctor will make very small openings in your eye wall and remove most of the vitreous from your eye with a suction tool.

[1] "Surgery for Refractive Errors," National Eye Institute (NEI), June 26, 2019. Available online. URL: www.nei.nih.gov/learn-about-eye-health/eye-conditions-and-diseases/refractive-errors/surgery-refractive-errors. Accessed August 5, 2024.

Depending on your treatment plan, your doctor may also:

- Use a laser or freeze treatment to reattach or repair your retina.
- Inject a bubble of air, other gas, or silicone oil into your eye to hold your retina in place.

Doctors can use numbing eye drops or shots to prevent pain during the surgery, or they can use general anesthesia to put you to sleep for the procedure. Before your vitrectomy surgery, discuss your anesthesia options with your doctor.

If you need vitrectomy in both eyes, the surgeries will be done separately. Your doctor can schedule surgery on the second eye after the first eye has recovered.

HOW LONG DOES IT TAKE TO RECOVER?

Most people go home the same day as the surgery. You will need someone to drive you home from the hospital.

Your eye may be swollen and red for several weeks after the surgery. While it is healing, you may experience some eye pain, and your vision may be blurrier than before the surgery. You will have follow-up appointments so your eye doctor can check your vision and ensure your eye is healing.

After the surgery, you will need to:

- **Wear an eye patch**. Usually for about a day.
- **Use eye drops**. To reduce swelling and prevent infections.
- **Avoid some activities**. Such as driving, intense exercise, and heavy lifting while your eye heals.
- **Take time off work**. Usually two to four weeks.

Ask your doctor when it is safe to return to work, start driving, and exercise again.

If the doctor puts a gas bubble in your eye, you will need to:

- Hold your head in a certain position for a few days to a few weeks to keep the gas bubble in the right spot.
- Avoid flying in an airplane or traveling to high altitudes while the bubble is in your eye.

Ask your doctor how long you need to follow these precautions after surgery.

Eventually, your eye will produce new fluid to replace the vitreous removed during the surgery. If the doctor used silicone oil during the procedure, you might need a second surgery to remove the oil.[1]

[1] "Vitrectomy," National Eye Institute (NEI), October 31, 2022. Available online. URL: www.nei.nih.gov/learn-about-eye-health/eye-conditions-and-diseases/retinal-detachment/vitrectomy. Accessed August 5, 2024.

Chapter 20 | Eye Devices for Anophthalmia and Microphthalmia

LIVING WITH ANOPHTHALMIA AND MICROPHTHALMIA

Anophthalmia and microphthalmia are eye conditions that people are born with. Anophthalmia occurs when a baby is born without one or both of its eyes, while microphthalmia refers to a baby's one or both eyes "being small." Both conditions are rare and can cause vision loss or blindness.

There is no treatment that can create a new eye or restore vision for people born with anophthalmia or microphthalmia. However, early treatment can help babies and children with these conditions grow and develop.[1]

EYE DEVICES

Conformers

Children with anophthalmia or microphthalmia may need to wear conformers (sometimes called "expanders")—plastic devices that help the eye socket grow to a normal size and shape. If your child needs a conformer, an ocularist (a specialist in eye devices) will create one that fits.

It is important for children who need conformers to start wearing them as early as possible. Because babies grow so fast, they must change to a larger conformer every few weeks or months until their growth slows down—usually around age 2.

---

[1] "Anophthalmia and Microphthalmia," National Eye Institute (NEI), November 15, 2023. Available online. URL: www.nei.nih.gov/learn-about-eye-health/eye-conditions-and-diseases/anophthalmia-and-microphthalmia. Accessed August 5, 2024.

Prosthetic Eyes

Once their eye socket reaches a normal size, children with anophthalmia or microphthalmia can wear a prosthetic eye—a device painted to look like their other eye. Children with microphthalmia can wear a type of prosthetic called a "scleral shell" that fits over their smaller eyes.

Prosthetic eyes can change the way children with anophthalmia or microphthalmia look. However, these devices do not restore vision.

Children usually get their first prosthetic eye between ages 1 and 2. As they grow and the shape of their faces changes, they will need a new prosthetic eye every few years. Most children must have their prosthetic eye replaced three to four times by age 10.

If your child has anophthalmia or microphthalmia, it is important to talk to all of their doctors about the best plan for their care. Babies with anophthalmia or microphthalmia also need early intervention and therapy—special services to help them grow and develop.[2]

[2] "Eye Devices for Anophthalmia and Microphthalmia," National Eye Institute (NEI), October 13, 2021. Available online. URL: www.nei.nih.gov/learn-about-eye-health/eye-conditions-and-diseases/anophthalmia-and-microphthalmia/eye-devices-anophthalmia-and-microphthalmia. Accessed August 5, 2024.

Chapter 21 | Preventing Vision Impairment and Blindness

Chapter Contents

Section 21.1 | Protecting Your Vision

COMMON EYE DISORDERS AND DISEASES

Some eye conditions can cause vision loss and even blindness. These include:

- cataracts, a clouding of the eye
- diabetic retinopathy (DR), which damages the blood vessels in the back of the eye
- glaucoma, damage to the optic nerve, often with increased eye pressure
- age-related macular degeneration (AMD), which gradually affects central vision

Other eye conditions, such as refractive errors, occur when the shape of your eye does not bend light correctly. These common problems can easily be corrected with glasses, contact lenses, or laser surgery. An estimated 11 million Americans aged 12 years and older could see better if they used corrective lenses or underwent eye surgery, if appropriate.

You can have a dilated eye exam regularly to check for common eye problems. Get the exam every 1–2 years if you:

- are over 60 years of age
- are African American and over 40 years of age
- have a family history of glaucoma

If you have diabetes or high blood pressure (HBP), ask your doctor how often you need an eye exam. Most people with diabetes or HBP need a dilated eye exam every year.

Although older adults tend to have more vision problems, preschoolers may not see as well as they can. The U.S. Preventive Services Task Force recommends that children have at least one eye exam between ages three and five years.

WAYS TO PROTECT YOUR VISION

- Get regular comprehensive dilated eye exams.
- Know your family's eye health history. It is important to know if anyone has been diagnosed with an eye disease or condition, as some are hereditary.

- Eat right to protect your sight. In particular, eat plenty of dark leafy greens such as spinach, kale, or collard greens, and fish that are high in omega-3 fatty acids such as salmon, albacore tuna, trout, and halibut.
- Maintain a healthy weight.
- Wear protective eyewear when playing sports or doing activities around the home, such as painting, yard work, and home repairs.
- Quit smoking or never start.
- Wear sunglasses that block at least 99 percent of ultraviolet A (UVA) and ultraviolet B (UVB) radiation.
- Wash your hands before taking out your contacts and clean your contact lenses properly to avoid infection.
- Practice workplace eye safety.

EYES AND OVERALL HEALTH

Taking care of your eyes may also benefit your overall health. Some health conditions, such as diabetes and HBP, can affect your eyes at the initial stage. An eye exam can inform you and your doctor if there are any underlying health conditions that need attention.

In addition to your comprehensive dilated eye exam, visit an eye care professional if you experience:

- decreased vision
- eye pain
- drainage or redness of the eye
- double vision
- floaters (tiny specks that appear to float before your eyes)
- circles (halos) around light sources
- flashes of light[1]

[1] "Taking Care of Your Eyes," Centers for Disease Control and Prevention (CDC), May 15, 2024. Available online. URL: www.cdc.gov/vision-health/prevention/taking-care-of-your-eyes.html. Accessed August 6, 2024.

Section 21.2 | Tips to Prevent Vision Loss

VISION HEALTH TIPS

Have a Comprehensive Eye Exam

You may not have any symptoms or eye problems, but visiting your eye care professional for a comprehensive dilated eye exam is the only way to be sure. Some people also do not realize they can see better with glasses or contact lenses. A dilated eye exam is the only way to detect some common eye diseases in their early stages, such as glaucoma, diabetic eye disease, and age-related macular degeneration (AMD). During a comprehensive dilated eye exam, your eye care professional places drops in your eyes to dilate them, allowing more light to enter the eye so your doctor can check for any signs of damage or disease.

Wear Protective Eyewear

Protective eyewear prevents eye injuries in the workplace, while playing sports, or during other activities that could cause damage. They include:

- safety glasses and goggles
- safety shields
- eye guards designed for specific activities

Most protective eyewear lenses are made of polycarbonate, which is 10 times stronger than other plastics. Many eye care providers and sporting goods stores sell protective eyewear. Employers are required to provide a safe work environment, which includes protective eyewear if needed.

Wear Sunglasses

Sunglasses are not just a fashion accessory; they are crucial for protecting your eyes from the sun's ultraviolet (UV) rays. When purchasing sunglasses, look for ones that block out 99–100 percent of both UV-A and UV-B radiation.

Give Your Eyes a Rest

If you spend much time at the computer or focusing on one thing, you might forget to blink. This can cause eye strain or fatigue. Employ the 20-20-20 rule: Every 20 minutes, look away about 20 feet in front of you for 20 seconds.

Clean Your Hands and Contact Lenses Properly

To avoid the risk of infection, always wash your hands thoroughly before putting in or taking out your contact lenses. Disinfect contact lenses as instructed and replace them as directed by your eye care professional.

MORE TIPS TO PREVENT VISION LOSS

Eat Right to Protect Your Sight

Eating a diet rich in fruits and vegetables helps keep your eyes healthy. You have heard that carrots are good for your eyes, but dark leafy greens such as spinach, kale, or collard greens also provide the vitamins and minerals your eyes need. Research also shows eye health benefits from fish high in omega-3 fatty acids, such as salmon, tuna, and halibut.

Maintain a Healthy Weight

Being overweight or obese increases the risk of developing type 2 diabetes and other chronic conditions that could damage your eyes. If you are having trouble maintaining a healthy weight, talk to your doctor.

Maintain Your Blood Sugar Levels

Ninety percent of blindness caused by diabetes is preventable. Ask your health-care team about goals to manage your A1C level (a measurement of blood sugar), blood pressure, and cholesterol. These are known as the "ABCs of diabetes."

Know Your Family's Eye Health History

Talk to your family members about their eye health history. It is important to know because some eye diseases or conditions are hereditary. This information will help determine if you are at higher risk for developing eye problems.

Quit Smoking or Do Not Start

Smoking is as harmful to your eyes as it is to the rest of your body. Research has linked smoking to an increased risk of developing:

- age-related macular degeneration
- cataracts
- optic nerve damage

All of these eye conditions can lead to blindness.[1]

[1] "Preventing Vision Loss," Centers for Disease Control and Prevention (CDC), May 15, 2024. Available online. URL: www.cdc.gov/vision-health/prevention. Accessed August 6, 2024.

Chapter 22 | Multidisciplinary Vision Rehabilitation

LIVING WITH VISUAL IMPAIRMENT

A visual impairment can make everyday activities such as driving or reading challenging. It is a condition that cannot be corrected with standard treatments such as glasses, contacts, medicine, or surgery. Millions of Americans live with some form of visual impairment.

Fortunately, vision rehabilitation services are available to assist individuals in maintaining their daily routines and continuing to enjoy their favorite activities.

WHAT IS VISION REHABILITATION?

Vision rehabilitation is designed to maximize the remaining vision of individuals with visual impairments and improve their quality of life (QOL). Various types of vision rehabilitation services are available, and consulting with your eye doctor or care team is an excellent first step in determining which services are best suited to your needs.

Examples of vision rehabilitation services include:

- employment and job training
- assistive products, such as specialized lighting and reading stands
- technology solutions, including magnifiers and screen readers
- training in daily living and independent living skills
- emotional support, such as counseling or support groups
- assistance with transportation and household tasks

WHO CAN BENEFIT FROM VISION REHABILITATION SERVICES?

Anyone with a visual impairment can benefit from vision rehabilitation services. These services provide essential skills and resources to help manage daily life and maintain independence.

HOW CAN YOU ACCESS VISION REHABILITATION SERVICES?

To access vision rehabilitation services, discuss your needs and goals with your eye doctor or care team. They can help identify the most suitable services for you and connect you with additional resources.

If you do not have an eye doctor, you can still access services independently. Here are several resources to help you find the necessary support:

- VisionAware's Directory of Services—offers a searchable directory by category and state (https://aphconnectcenter.org).
- Rehabilitation Services Administration's State Vocational Rehabilitation Agency Directory—lists state-specific resources (https://rsa.ed.gov/about/states).
- American Optometric Association's Eye Doctor Directory—you can refine your search by selecting specialists in low vision and vision rehabilitation (www.aoa.org/healthy-eyes/find-a-doctor?sso=y).
- American Academy of Ophthalmology's Ophthalmologist Directory—you can filter by the "vision rehab" subspecialty (https://secure.aao.org/aao/find-ophthalmologist).

Additional resources for support include:

- American Academy of Ophthalmology's Resources for People with Low Vision (www.aao.org/eye-health/diseases/low-vision-resources).
- American Optometric Association's Vision Rehabilitation Resources (www.aoa.org/healthy-eyes/caring-for-your-eyes/low-vision-and-vision-rehab?sso=y).

- Hadley's Daily Living Workshops, including a series on cooking safely with a visual impairment (https://hadleyhelps.org/learn?topic_id=12).
- Lighthouse Guild's Tele-Support Groups (https://lighthouseguild.org/support-services/telesupport-groups).
- Prevent Blindness' Resources for Living Well with Low Vision (https://lowvision.preventblindness.org).
- The Vision Council's Low Vision Resources (https://thevisioncouncilfoundation.org/eye-care-and-eye-health/low-vision).

Finding the right vision rehabilitation services and supports may take time, but the effort is well worth it to enhance your QOL and maintain your independence.[1]

LOW VISION AND BLINDNESS REHABILITATION RESEARCH

The National Eye Institute (NEI) supports extensive research to:

- investigate multisensory processes, cross-modal plasticity, and cortical reorganization in visually impaired individuals
- increase understanding of different types of visual impairment in complex or applied settings
- create and validate vision tests relevant for daily living tasks and rehabilitative goals
- design mobile assistive devices and navigation resources to enhance wayfinding
- develop new adaptive technologies to improve access to Internet, print, graphic displays, and educational resources
- characterize acceptable levels of visual enhancement using aids and prosthetics

---

[1] "Vision Rehabilitation," National Eye Institute (NEI), July 24, 2023. Available online. URL: www.nei.nih.gov/learn-about-eye-health/vision-rehabilitation. Accessed August 6, 2024.

- identify comorbidities that interact with vision impairment and their effect on rehabilitation needs and outcomes
- develop and test visual rehabilitation models and training paradigms

This research aims to advance knowledge and technology, improving the lives of those with visual impairments through more effective rehabilitation methods and tools.[2]

[2] "Low Vision and Blindness Rehabilitation," National Eye Institute (NEI), August 3, 2021. Available online. URL: www.nei.nih.gov/grants-and-training/funding-opportunities/programs-and-research-priorities/low-vision-and-blindness-rehabilitation. Accessed August 6, 2024.

Chapter 23 | Enhancing Vision: Interventions and Innovations

OVERVIEW OF EFFECTIVE MEDICAL INTERVENTIONS

Some medical interventions, including laser photocoagulation, vitreous surgery, and cataract surgery with lens implantation, are effective in preventing blindness and/or improving vision among certain indicated patients. However, rehabilitation for individuals with low vision focuses on services for those without medical options.

ASSISTIVE DEVICES AND THEIR EFFECT

The rehabilitation literature outside the field of vision impairment indicates that the use of assistive devices can have positive effects. Individuals with nonvision disabilities who use such devices can become more independent, and the devices can mitigate the effects of disabilities. For people with low vision, a variety of optical and electronic aids may help to carry out everyday activities. Generally, optical aids enhance vision mainly through magnification or vision field enhancement.

TRAINING AND USAGE OF OPTICAL DEVICES

A two-year study of veterans who received low vision devices from the U.S. Department of Veterans Affairs (VA) found that subjects reported the devices to be beneficial, and they used them for a variety of tasks. The selection of aids depends on the underlying cause of the visual disability, personal preference, and other factors. A single device will usually not meet the needs of all tasks likely to be encountered. Categories of optical devices used in the field of low vision rehabilitation include:

- high-plus spectacles
- hand-held magnifiers

- magnification of relative distance, relative size, angular, and projection
- stand magnifiers
- telescopes
- video magnifiers (closed-circuit television)
- absorptive lenses
- field-expanding devices

According to the American Occupational Therapy Association, training in the use of optical devices is needed for optimal effectiveness. When 125 patients received simple low-vision aids with an emphasis on training in their use, self-reported satisfaction and use of the aids were higher compared to patients who received the aids without training. Instruction in eccentric viewing (utilizing a portion of the peripheral retina for tasks such as reading and mobility) and page-orientation techniques may also be useful. Alternative methods of reading include Braille (or electronic Braille displays), electronic reading devices that enable printed text to be synthesized into speech, audiotapes, and reader services. It is unclear how frequently these alternative methods are used; Lighthouse International estimates that fewer than 10 percent of the legally blind in the United States read Braille.

NONOPTICAL DEVICES AND TECHNIQUES

It is notable that training is not limited to practical device use or daily living skills. Training may also occur at the basic perceptual level. For example, peripheral vision training can aim to compensate for lost central vision. The effectiveness of the different categories of training is not yet known. However, there is a consensus among the expert advisors for this study that training is critical.

Nonoptical devices and techniques that can help improve the daily functioning of these individuals include:

- relative-size techniques (accessibility of these has increased with the increased availability of computers)
- lighting, glare, contrast, and color modification
- ergonomic posture and positioning

- written communication assistive technologies
- medical management
- mobility
- sensory substitution

Other techniques to improve the use of residual vision include lighting optimization and contrast enhancement. Although illumination levels will be based on personal preference, there are some general guidelines. For example, the light for detailed close work is best provided when it is directed from behind the person, decreasing potential glare. Also, directional lighting (e.g., with a gooseneck lamp) is useful for lighting a task without shining light into the person's eyes. Dimmer switches allow for varying levels of illumination depending on the task at hand. Halogen lamps, which provide more intense illumination, are helpful for individuals with age-related macular degeneration (AMD). Contrast enhancement can be accomplished by adequate lighting or electronic magnifiers and proper selection of writing and reading materials (e.g., bold-print media, black ink on white paper).

ORIENTATION AND MOBILITY SYSTEMS

The four most common systems used to enhance orientation and mobility skills are functional vision, a human guide, a long cane, and a dog guide. Other techniques include "walking along," which refers to following an environmental feature, such as a curb. Electronic travel aids (ETAs), which emit light or sound, may be included in the list of orientation and mobility systems. However, there are several obstacles to greater use of ETAs. They are currently expensive, require significant training, and may provide insufficient amounts of information to the user (e.g., they often cannot detect changes in surface levels such as a curb). Electronic aids that use digital and satellite navigation intended for orientation in larger spaces have not yet been widely adopted. Typically, individuals use functional vision and one of the other systems to enhance their orientation and mobility skills, or they use a system (such as a human guide) selectively. It is important to point out that the evidence base for orientation and mobility training is weak. There has been very little research on the short- or long-term effectiveness of orientation and mobility techniques or on the degree of safety they offer.

INFLUENCE OF TECHNOLOGICAL ADVANCES

There is limited, though generally inconclusive, evidence differentiating the effectiveness of some low-technology interventions. For example, half-field eye patching for unilateral spatial neglect has been shown in a randomized controlled trial (RCT) involving 22 subjects to significantly improve functioning to a greater extent than monocular patching. The effectiveness of a given device may differ depending on the cause of low vision. For example, persons with restricted visual fields are least served by available devices, and devices for increasing field awareness are ineffective.

Whether for society at large or for people with low vision in particular, technological advances have both undesirable and desirable effects. Negative outcomes occur when technologies raise barriers to entry into the workforce by eliminating low-skilled jobs, changing the nature of work, or when individuals may benefit from technology but lack access to it. One example of a negative influence of advanced technology on people with low vision is the widespread use of graphic user interface (GUI) software for computing. Whereas computers based on DOS were relatively easy to modify for use by the visually impaired, Windows® or other graphic systems are difficult to convert into audio or Braille text. In addition, as telecommunications become more oriented to visual media, barriers will be created for the visually impaired. On the other hand, the use of voice in technological devices will increase access, allowing the visually impaired to use telecommunications even for the interpretation of face-to-face interaction. This is possible due to advances in electronics and voice technology, and network-based services that translate information across communication modes (e.g., voice descriptions of visual information). Such technological promise notwithstanding, it is likely to be necessary to demonstrate the effectiveness of these advances for the visually impaired to secure third-party payment for them, where applicable.

SELECTION AND MATCHING OF VISION AIDS

Many evolving optical and nonoptical aids and techniques are available to enhance the daily functioning of individuals with vision impairment. The literature highlights the importance of the user-technology interface and emphasizes the importance of matching the device and technique to the needs of the individual. In addition to clinical medical evaluation, this includes consideration of social, psychological, familial, financial, and other factors. Technical factors to be considered in selecting optical devices include power, working distance, working space, field of view, light, focal length, depth of field, and light transmission. However, despite the availability of these technologies and the consensus regarding the need to match them to user-specific needs, there is no clear-cut evidence concerning which devices and techniques are beneficial to people with particular impairments.[1]

[1] Agency for Healthcare Research and Quality (AHRQ), "Vision Rehabilitation: Care and Benefit Plan Models: Literature Review," U.S. Department of Health and Human Services (HHS), September 2012. Available online. URL: www.ahrq.gov/prevention/resources/vision/resources/vision2.html. Accessed August 6, 2024.

Chapter 24 | Innovations in Technology for Low Vision and Blindness

The National Eye Institute (NEI), part of the National Institutes of Health (NIH), highlights new technologies and tools being developed to assist the 4.1 million Americans living with low vision or blindness. These innovations aim to simplify daily tasks for those with vision loss, such as navigating office buildings or crossing streets. Many innovations leverage computer vision, a technology that enables computers to recognize and interpret a complex assortment of images, objects, and behaviors in their environment.

Low vision means that even with glasses, contact lenses, medicine, or surgery, individuals find everyday tasks challenging. This condition can affect many aspects of life, from walking in crowded places to reading or preparing meals, explained Cheri Wiggs, PhD, program director, NEI. The necessary tools vary based on the degree and type of vision loss. For instance, glaucoma causes loss of peripheral vision, complicating walking or driving. Conversely, age-related macular degeneration affects central vision, hindering activities such as reading.

Here is a look at a few NEI-funded technologies under development that aim to lessen the effect of low vision and blindness.

CO-ROBOTIC CANE

Indoor navigation poses a significant challenge for individuals with low vision or blindness. While Global Positioning System (GPS)-based devices can guide users to a general location, such as a building, they are less helpful in locating specific rooms, explained Cang

Ye, PhD, University of Arkansas at Little Rock. Ye has developed a co-robotic cane that provides feedback about the user's surrounding environment. This prototype features a computerized 3D camera to visualize the environment for the user and a motorized roller tip that propels the cane toward a desired location. The user can issue verbal commands through a microphone, which a speech recognition system interprets, providing guidance through a wireless earpiece. The cane's compact computer stores preloaded floor plans and can download new ones via Wi-Fi upon entering a building. It analyzes 3D information in real time, alerting the user to hallways and stairs, and gauges the user's location by comparing successive images captured by the camera. In addition to NEI support, Ye recently received a grant from the NIH's Coulter College Commercializing Innovation Program to explore the commercialization of this robotic cane.

ROBOTIC GLOVE FOR DETECTING DOOR HANDLES AND OBJECTS

While developing the co-robotic cane, Ye identified another challenge: navigating closed doorways. "Finding the door knob or handle and opening the door significantly slows you down," he said. To assist users with locating and grasping small objects more quickly, he designed a fingerless glove equipped with a camera and a speech recognition system. This glove guides the user's hand to objects such as door handles, mugs, or bottles of water through tactile prompts. "Directing the hand left or right is straightforward," Ye noted. "An actuator on the thumb's surface facilitates this in an intuitive and natural manner." The glove also features a novel hybrid tactile system, developed by Ye's colleague Yantao Shen, PhD, University of Nevada, Reno, which uses mechanical and electrical stimuli to simulate a sense of touch.

SMARTPHONE CROSSWALK APP

Street crossings are particularly hazardous for those with low vision. To address this, James Coughlan, PhD, and his team at the Smith-Kettlewell Eye Research Institute developed a smartphone app that provides auditory prompts to help users find the safest crossing locations and stay within crosswalks. The app combines GPS, computer vision, and a geographic information system (GIS) to overcome each technology's limitations and provide comprehensive guidance at intersections.

CAMIO SYSTEM FOR EXPLORING OBJECTS NATURALLY

The CamIO system, also developed by Coughlan, enables visually impaired students to explore objects like a 3D anatomical heart model or read the display on devices such as glucose monitors through auditory feedback. This low-cost system, connected to a laptop, provides real-time audio feedback as the user interacts with various objects, from maps to digital displays. Coughlan plans to develop a smartphone app version of CamIO, with the current laptop software available for free download.

HIGH-POWERED PRISMS AND PERISCOPES FOR SEVERE TUNNEL VISION

Eli Peli, OD, Schepens Eye Research Institute in Boston, has designed lenses made of adjacent 1-millimeter-wide prisms to expand the visual field for people with severe peripheral vision loss due to conditions such as retinitis pigmentosa and glaucoma. To achieve a wider field of view, Peli and his team use a periscope-like concept with nonparallel mirrors to develop a prototype that provides a 45-degree visual field, aiming for a cosmetically acceptable version that could be incorporated into eyeglasses.

These technologies demonstrate significant advancements in aiding individuals with low vision or blindness, enhancing their ability to navigate and interact with their environment more effectively.[1]

[1] "Five Innovations Harness New Technologies for People with Visual Impairment, Blindness," National Eye Institute (NEI), February 3, 2017. Available online. URL: www.nei.nih.gov/about/news-and-events/news/five-innovations-harness-new-technologies-people-visual-impairment-blindness. Accessed August 5, 2024.

Chapter 25 | Braille Services

Braille services play a vital role in facilitating access to information and communication for individuals with blindness or visual impairment. In the early 1800s, Charles Barbier, an artillery captain in Napoleon Bonaparte's French army, created a system to read combat messages safely at night. This system was known as "night writing." The system used 12-dot cells comprising two columns and six rows overall impressed onto paper so they are raised. A combination of dots represented a phonetic sound or a letter. Louis Braille, a French educator, who was blinded at the age of three after an eye injury, modified Charles Barbier's night writing system. He used 6 dots because the 12-dot system was challenging to feel by fingertip. After years of work, in 1824, this came to be known as the "braille system," named after the inventor, comprising 63 characters. Braille is used today with several modifications that have made reading more accessible for individuals with blindness or visual impairment.

THE BRAILLE ALPHABET

The braille alphabet consists of characters represented by six dots in one cell, arranged in two columns and three rows. To read braille, users move their fingertips across a series of raised dots arranged in a specific pattern. Each set of raised dots represents a letter. The system has been modified so that commonly used words have separate representations. Numbers are represented in correspondence to the letter, meaning the sign for the number one is the letter A, two is the letter B, and so on.

BRAILLE EDUCATION

Schools and organizations offer braille instruction to individuals of all ages, teaching them how to read and write in braille. This education may also include orientation and mobility training to enhance independent living skills. These institutions specialize in educating students who are blind or visually impaired, offering comprehensive braille instruction programs throughout a student's academic journey, from elementary to high school or even college-preparatory levels.

TYPES OF BRAILLE SERVICES

Braille exists in two forms: grade 1 (alphabetic or non-contracted braille) and grade 2 (contracted braille). Grade 1 braille substitutes standard letters with braille codes. Grade 2 braille is a shorthand system where a single pattern represents frequent combinations of letters or words. Grade 2 braille makes reading faster and more efficient. With advancements in technology, various devices have been designed to read and write content through braille. Some of them include:

- **Braille transcription**. This converts printed materials such as textbooks, articles, or other resources into braille format using specialized software or manual transcription. Braille transcriptionists ensure accuracy and readability by adhering to braille standards and guidelines.
- **Braille printing**. Once transcribed, braille documents can be embossed onto paper using braille printers. These printers create raised dots that can be felt with the fingertips, allowing individuals with visual impairment to read the text through touch.
- **Braille displays**. Electronic braille displays convert digital text into braille output, providing real-time access to information from computers, smartphones, and other devices. These displays use refreshable braille cells, which are small mechanical elements that move up and down to form braille characters as the user navigates through content. Each cell typically represents one braille character, and as the user scrolls or reads, the cells dynamically change to display new text, allowing for continuous access to digital information in braille format.
- **Notetaker**. Originally used for taking notes and storing phone numbers in braille, Notetakers have been modified and can now be used for various purposes such as web browsing, writing, and reading books.

IMPORTANCE OF BRAILLE SERVICES

Braille services facilitate access to information, enabling equal opportunities for individuals who are blind or visually impaired.

- **Accessibility**. Braille services promote inclusivity by making printed materials accessible to individuals with visual impairment. This includes books, documents, labels, and signage in various settings such as schools, libraries, workplaces, and public spaces.
- **Independence**. Learning braille empowers individuals to access information independently, enhancing their educational and employment opportunities. It fosters self-sufficiency and confidence in navigating the world around them.
- **Literacy**. Braille literacy is crucial for the intellectual development and academic success of individuals with blindness and visual impairment. It enables them to engage with written material at the same level as their sighted peers, overcoming impediments to learning.

Braille remains an essential tool for individuals with visual impairment to access information. Technological advancements have designed various devices to read, write, and provide real-time access to information from computers, smartphones, and other devices, making it easier for individuals with visual impairment to comprehend written content.

References

"About Braille," National Library Service (NLS), July 9, 2017. Available online. URL: www.loc.gov/nls/services-and-resources/informational-publications/about-braille. Accessed August 7, 2024.

"Description and History of Braille," American Council of the Blind (ACB), January 31, 2001. Available online. URL: www.acb.org/history-of-braille. Accessed August 7, 2024.

"How to Read and Write Braille," IOWA Department for the Blind, July 1, 2023. Available online. URL: https://blind.iowa.gov/educators/how-read-and-write-braille. Accessed August 7, 2024.

"What Is Braille?" American Foundation for the Blind (AFB), March 18, 2015. Available online. URL: www.afb.org/blindness-and-low-vision/braille/what-braille. Accessed August 7, 2024.

Part 4 | **Disability Support for Vision Impairment**

Chapter 26 | **Mobility Aids for People with Visual Impairments**

Chapter Contents

Section 26.1 | Robotic Cane with 3D Camera

INTRODUCTION TO THE ROBOTIC CANE

Equipped with a color 3D camera, an inertial measurement sensor, and its own onboard computer, a newly improved robotic cane could offer blind and visually impaired users a new way to navigate indoors. When paired with a building's architectural drawing, the device can accurately guide a user to a desired location with sensory and auditory cues, while simultaneously helping the user avoid obstacles such as boxes, furniture, and overhangs. The development of the device was co-funded by the National Institutes of Health's (NIH) National Eye Institute (NEI) and the National Institute of Biomedical Imaging and Bioengineering (NIBIB). Details of the updated design were published in the journal *IEEE/CAA Journal of Automatica Sinica.*

ADVANCEMENTS IN NAVIGATION TECHNOLOGY

"Many people in the visually impaired community consider the white cane to be their best and most functional navigational tool, despite it being century-old technology," said Cang Ye, PhD, lead author of the study and professor of computer science at the College of Engineering at the Virginia Commonwealth University, Richmond. "For sighted people, technologies like GPS-based applications have revolutionized navigation. We're interested in creating a device that closes many of the gaps in functionality for white cane users."

CHALLENGES IN INDOOR NAVIGATION

While there are cellphone-based applications that can provide navigation assistance—helping users with blindness stay within crosswalks, for example—large spaces inside buildings are a major challenge, especially when those spaces are unfamiliar. Earlier versions of Ye's robotic cane began tackling this problem by incorporating building floorplans; the user could tell the cane where he or she wished to go, and the cane—through a combination of auditory cues and a robotic rolling tip—could guide the user to their destination. However, when used over long distances, the inaccuracies in the user's location could build up, eventually leaving the user at an incorrect location.

INTEGRATION OF DEPTH CAMERA TECHNOLOGY

To help correct this issue, Ye and colleagues have added a color depth camera to the system. Using infrared light, much like a mobile phone's front-facing camera, the system can determine the distance between the cane and other physical objects, including the floor, features such as doorways and walls, as well as furniture and other obstacles. Using this information, along with data from an inertial sensor, the cane's onboard computer can map the user's precise location to the existing architectural drawing or floorplan, while also alerting the user to obstacles in their path.

PRECISION AND SAFETY FEATURES

"While some cell phone apps can give people auditory navigation instructions, when going around a corner for example, how do you know you've turned just the right amount?" said Ye. "The rolling tip on our robotic cane can guide you to turn at just the right point and exactly the right number of degrees, whether it's 15 degrees or 90. This version can also alert you to overhanging obstacles, which a standard white cane cannot."

FUTURE IMPROVEMENTS AND MARKET READINESS

There are still a few kinks to be worked out before the system will be market-ready—it is still too heavy for regular use, for example, and Ye's team is looking for a way to slim down the device. Nevertheless, with the ability to easily switch between its automated mode and a simpler, non-robotic "white cane mode," Ye believes this device could provide a key independence tool for the blind and visually impaired, without losing the characteristics of the white cane that have stood the test of time.[1]

---

[1] "NIH-Funded Modern 'White Cane' Brings Navigation Assistance to the 21st Century," National Eye Institute (NEI), September 8, 2021. Available online. URL: www.nei.nih.gov/about/news-and-events/news/nih-funded-modern-white-cane-brings-navigation-assistance-21st-century. Accessed August 5, 2024.

Section 26.2 | Guide Dogs

Beginning on March 15, 2011, only dogs are recognized as service animals under titles II and III of the Americans with Disabilities Act (ADA). A service animal is a dog that is individually trained to do work or perform tasks for a person with a disability. Generally, title II and title III entities must permit service animals to accompany people with disabilities in all areas where members of the public are allowed to go.

HOW "SERVICE ANIMAL" IS DEFINED

Service animals are defined as dogs that are individually trained to do work or perform tasks for people with disabilities. Examples of such work or tasks include:

- guiding people who are blind
- alerting people who are deaf
- pulling a wheelchair
- alerting and protecting a person who is having a seizure
- reminding a person with mental illness to take prescribed medications
- calming a person with posttraumatic stress disorder (PTSD) during an anxiety attack

Service animals are working animals, not pets. The work or task a dog has been trained to provide must be directly related to the person's disability. Dogs whose sole function is to provide comfort or emotional support do not qualify as service animals under the ADA.

INQUIRIES, EXCLUSIONS, CHARGES, AND OTHER SPECIFIC RULES RELATED TO SERVICE ANIMALS

When it is not obvious what service an animal provides, only limited inquiries are allowed. Staff may ask two questions:

1. Is the dog a service animal required because of a disability?
2. What work or task has the dog been trained to perform?

Staff cannot ask about the person's disability, require medical documentation, require a special identification card or training documentation for the dog, or ask that the dog demonstrate its ability to perform the work or task.

Allergies and fear of dogs are not valid reasons for denying access or refusing service to people using service animals. When a person who is allergic to dog dander and a person who uses a service animal must spend time in the same room or facility, they both should be accommodated by assigning them, if possible, to different locations within the room or different rooms in the facility.

A person with a disability cannot be asked to remove his service animal from the premises unless:

- the dog is out of control, and the handler does not take effective action to control it
- the dog is not housebroken

When there is a legitimate reason to ask that a service animal be removed, staff must offer the person with the disability the opportunity to obtain goods or services without the animal's presence.

Establishments that sell or prepare food must generally allow service animals in public areas even if state or local health codes prohibit animals on the premises.

People with disabilities who use service animals cannot be isolated from other patrons, treated less favorably than other patrons, or charged fees that are not charged to other patrons without animals. In addition, if a business requires a deposit or fee to be paid by patrons with pets, it must waive the charge for service animals.

If a business such as a hotel normally charges guests for damage that they cause, a customer with a disability may also be charged for damage caused by himself or his service animal.

Staff are not required to provide care for or supervision of a service animal.[1]

[1] ADA.gov, "ADA Requirements: Service Animals," U.S. Department of Justice (DOJ), February 28, 2020. Available online. URL: www.ada.gov/resources/service-animals-2010-requirements. Accessed August 7, 2024.

EXAMPLES OF SERVICE ANIMAL TASKS

- A person who uses a wheelchair may have a dog that is trained to retrieve objects for them.
- A person with depression may have a dog that is trained to perform a task to remind them to take their medication.
- A person with PTSD may have a dog that is trained to lick their hand to alert them to an oncoming panic attack.
- A person who has epilepsy may have a dog that is trained to detect the onset of a seizure and then help the person remain safe during the seizure.

WHERE SERVICE ANIMALS CAN GO

Generally, service animals are allowed to be with their person, even in places that do not allow pets. For example, service dogs can go into:

- restaurants
- shops
- hospitals
- schools
- hotels

Example. A restaurant offers indoor and outdoor seating. A woman arrives with her service dog and asks to sit inside. The restaurant cannot require the woman to dine outside because of her service dog.

The ADA also applies to certain types of housing, including:

- housing at public and private universities
- public housing programs run by state, county, and city governments
- emergency shelters

ASKING IF A DOG IS A SERVICE ANIMAL

If you are working at a business or state/local government facility, and it is unclear to you whether someone's dog is a service dog, you may ask for certain information using two questions:

- Is the dog a service animal required because of a disability?
- What work or task has the dog been trained to perform?

You are not allowed to:

- request any documentation that the dog is registered, licensed, or certified as a service animal
- require that the dog demonstrate its task, or inquire about the nature of the person's disability

Because service animals are not required to wear vests, a dog that is wearing a vest is not necessarily a service animal. The dog still needs to be trained to perform a task for a person with a disability to be a service animal.

WHEN A SERVICE ANIMAL CAN BE KEPT OUT

A business or state/local government does not need to allow a service animal if the dog's presence fundamentally alters the nature of the goods, services, programs, or activities provided to the public.

ASKING SOMEONE TO REMOVE THEIR SERVICE ANIMAL

A business or state/local government can ask someone to remove their service animal if the dog is:

- not housebroken
- out of control, and the person cannot get the dog under control

STATE AND LOCAL LAWS

State/local governments can:

- require service dogs to be licensed and vaccinated if all dogs are required to be licensed and vaccinated
- offer voluntary service dog registration programs

State/local governments cannot:

- require certification or registration of service dogs
- ban a service dog based on its breed[2]

---

[2] ADA.gov, "Service Animals," U.S. Department of Justice (DOJ), June 17, 2021. Available online. URL: www.ada.gov/topics/service-animals. Accessed August 7, 2024.

Chapter 27 | **Transportation Guide for People with Vision Impairment**

Chapter Contents

Section 27.1 | Transport for People with Vision Loss

There are several systems designed to help overcome the barriers faced by people with visual impairments in day-to-day life. Examples include large tactile print maps, accessible Global Positioning System (GPS), geographic information system (GIS), variable message signs, remote infrared audible signs (RIAS), real-time passenger information systems, vehicle "destination" and "next stop" signs, accessible ticket machines, and detectable warning surfaces.

ADDRESSING BARRIERS WITH TECHNOLOGY

One example of a barrier faced by people with visual impairments is when construction blocks a pedestrian right-of-way and forces a change of direction for a traveler. It is important to know what to do at that point, and a speaking sign would aid someone with a visual impairment in this situation.

TRIP CHAIN CHALLENGES

During a typical trip, a person with a visual impairment faces a number of challenges. A trip can be considered a chain of activities, and any broken link in the chain can significantly delay a trip. Delays can bring about frustration and prevent a traveler from attempting the trip a second time.

When faced with an unfamiliar trip on a public transit system, the chain can be seen as the following sequence of events: travelers must arrive at the beginning of their journey and identify that they are at the correct place; they must locate a fare machine and pay; they need to find the correct location for boarding the vehicle in a station; once underway, they need to identify the correct stop; and finally, they need to exit the vehicle and the transit system. Each step is made difficult for travelers with visual impairment because of a lack of accessible communication.

MAPPING CLARITY

Maps are useful tools for travel planning; however, standard on-screen mapping, such as Google Maps, presents several challenges for those with impairments. For example, zooming in will increase the width of a street, but it does not increase the font size.

With these limitations in mind, a selection of parameters has been identified as important to low-vision users of on-screen maps: font size, font style, color choice for text, line thickness for streets, overall color and contrast, and quality of the information displayed. If users were offered a customization tool, they would be able to set up their page according to personal preference.

SIGNS THAT TALK: REMOTE INFRARED AUDIBLE SIGNS

One useful tool to aid a visually impaired person in getting around is RIAS, a system that labels the environment so people who cannot read printed signs still have access to that information. A receiver on the unit converts a transmitted infrared signal into a voice message.

A user can scan the area for infrared transmitter labeling on many things, including bus stops, ticket machines, boarding areas, restrooms, elevators, and stairs. Its other functionality includes detecting and providing information on wait times, destination information, and pedestrian crossings. The directional system means that as a user walks in the direction of a particular sign, the message becomes clearer and louder—RIAS only detects the strongest signal a user is pointing toward.

An example of another RIAS application could be a person approaching an intersection: the system could provide a message about the crossing, such as whether it is a one-way street or has a diagonal crosswalk. The narrow-beam signal could also tell one pedestrian to wait and inform another when they are in the crosswalk. RIAS can also be used for museum exhibit information, and it is in use in many applications outside the United States, including the Oslo opera house, and locations in Japan, Italy, and Canada.

CONVERGENT TECHNOLOGY

There are many other convergent technologies involved with RIAS. For example, a bus stop system installed in Italy has implemented RIAS developments with mobile communications technology and features a wireless, solar-powered connection providing bus information to travelers.

Other technologies that RIAS can interact with include smartphones, which feature many built-in useful features, such as a keyboard and touch screen. They also offer several communication options including Wi-Fi and Bluetooth. For example, with access to the wireless Web community, mobile RIAS could send a request via Bluetooth to retrieve information; a mobile phone could send that request to a server, receive a reply from the server, and then communicate that back to the handset via Bluetooth. The handset can then provide that information and receive speech input to navigate menu options.[1]

Section 27.2 | Guide to Paratransit Systems

HOW PARATRANSIT ELIGIBILITY IS DETERMINED

Disability alone does not determine paratransit eligibility; the decision is based on the applicant's functional ability to use the fixed-route bus and is not a medical decision. The Department of Transportation (DOT) Americans with Disabilities Act (ADA) regulations in Appendix D to 49 C.F.R. Section 37.125 explain:

The substantive eligibility process is not aimed at making a medical or diagnostic determination. While evaluation by a physician (or professionals in rehabilitation or other relevant fields) may be used as part of the process, a diagnosis of a disability is not dispositive. What is needed is a determination of whether, as a practical matter, the individual can use fixed route transit in his or her own circumstances.

Transit agencies devise the specifics of their individual eligibility processes with input from the communities they serve. The DOT ADA regulations in Section 37.125 set only broad requirements that all agencies must incorporate, such as written notification of eligibility decisions and an opportunity for an appeal.

---

[1] "Technological Innovations in Transportation for People with Disabilities," U.S. Department of Transportation (DOT), February 23, 2011. Available online. URL: https://highways.dot.gov/media/5066. Accessed August 7, 2024.

USING PARATRANSIT SERVICE WHILE TRAVELING

If an individual is eligible for ADA paratransit in their place of residence, they have the right to use paratransit service in a city where they are traveling. Under DOT ADA regulations at 49 C.F.R. Section 37.127, each public entity required to provide complementary paratransit service must make the service available to visitors as provided under the section. The transit entity must provide service to visitors who present documentation that they are ADA paratransit eligible in the jurisdiction in which they reside, under the criteria of 49 C.F.R. Section 37.125. If a visitor with a disability does not present such documentation, the transit entity may require documentation of the individual's place of residence and of his or her disability, if the disability is not apparent. A transit operator is not required to provide service to a visitor for more than 21 days during any 365-day period; after that, the visitor may be required to apply for eligibility through the same processes established for residents under 49 C.F.R. Section 37.125.

APPEALING A TRANSIT AGENCY'S DECISION

Under DOT ADA regulations at 49 C.F.R. Section 37.125(g), transit operators must "establish an administrative appeal process through which individuals who are denied eligibility can obtain review of the denial." The transit operator may require that any appeal be filed within 60 days of the denial of an application. The appeal process must include an opportunity for the applicant to be heard and to present information and arguments. Decisions regarding the appeal cannot be made by anyone who was involved in the initial decision to deny eligibility. The transit operator must provide the individual with written notification of its decision and its reasons. The transit operator is not required to provide paratransit service while the appeal is under consideration; however, if a decision has not been made within 30 days of the completion of the appeal process, the operator must provide paratransit service from that time until and unless a decision to deny the appeal is issued.

ACCOMPANIMENT BY INDIVIDUALS

Under DOT ADA regulations at 49 C.F.R. Section 37.123(f), transit entities must permit one person to accompany the paratransit-eligible individual. Additional persons accompanying the eligible individual are to be served on a space-available basis to prevent displacement of other ADA paratransit eligible individuals. The transit provider may not limit who the companion may be; the companion may be a family member, friend, business associate, and so on. The transit authority may require that the eligible individual reserve a space for the companion when reserving his or her own ride. A personal care attendant (PCA), someone designated or employed to assist the eligible individual, may always ride with the eligible individual. The transit entity may require that the eligible individual reserve a space for the PCA when reserving the trip. If there is a PCA on the trip, the eligible individual may still bring a companion, as well as additional companions on a space-available basis. To be considered as "accompanying" the eligible individual, a companion must have the same origin and destination points as the eligible individual.

NUMBER OF DESTINATIONS OR TRIP LEGS

There is no limit on how many destinations or legs of a trip a paratransit rider may request in a given day. Paratransit providers must provide all eligible requested trips, not just trips to and from a single location. A person may take as many individual legs of a trip in a day as their schedule allows (factoring in pickup windows and time to complete their business), just as a fixed route user may take as many trips as he or she desires. For example, just as a person may take a fixed route from their home to work, then from work to an appointment, and then home again, so should a paratransit rider be able to. Each leg may be separately scheduled (i.e., paratransit providers are not required to wait while a passenger runs into the post office, just as a fixed route user would be required to wait for the next bus).[1]

[1] "Frequently Asked Questions," U.S. Department of Transportation (DOT), August 21, 2015. Available online. URL: www.transit.dot.gov/regulations-and-guidance/civil-rights-ada/frequently-asked-questions#1. Accessed August 7, 2024.

Chapter 28 | **Disability Employment Rights**

Chapter Contents

Section 28.1 | Visual Disabilities in the Workplace and the Americans with Disabilities Act

The Americans with Disabilities Act (ADA) applies to job applicants and employees with visual disabilities. Key aspects include the following:

- When an employer may ask an applicant or employee questions about vision impairment and how an employer should treat voluntary disclosures.
- What types of reasonable accommodations applicants or employees with visual disabilities may need.
- How an employer should handle safety concerns about applicants and employees with visual disabilities.
- How an employer can ensure that no employee is harassed because of a visual disability.

The U.S. Equal Employment Opportunity Commission (EEOC) enforces and provides leadership and guidance on the employment provisions of the ADA, a federal law prohibiting discrimination against qualified individuals with disabilities. Under the ADA, individuals with disabilities include those who have "a physical or mental impairment that substantially limits one or more major life activities," have a record (or history) of such an impairment, or are subject to an adverse action "because of an actual or perceived physical or mental impairment whether the impairment limits or is perceived to limit a major life activity."

Title I, the employment provision of the ADA, covers employment by private employers with 15 or more employees, as well as state and local government employers. Section 501 of the Rehabilitation Act of 1973 (Rehabilitation Act) provides similar protections to federal applicants and employees. In addition, most states have their own laws prohibiting employment discrimination based on disability. Some of these state laws may apply to smaller employers and may provide protections in addition to those available under the ADA.

GENERAL INFORMATION ABOUT VISION IMPAIRMENTS

In 2022, the U.S. Centers for Disease Control and Prevention's (CDC) National Health Interview Survey found that approximately 18.4 percent of all U.S. adults are blind or have "some" or "a lot" of difficulty seeing, even when wearing corrective lenses.

Many factors can affect an individual's vision, including the physiology of the eye and differences in how the brain interprets messages from the eye. Vision impairments can start or occur at any time in life. Some major causes of blindness and low vision in U.S. adults are eye diseases, including diabetic retinopathy (DR), macular degeneration, cataracts, and glaucoma. Other common eye conditions in the United States include amblyopia (the brain favoring one eye over the other) and strabismus (differences in the alignment of the eyes), although many other conditions exist. Some individuals experience eye injury, burns, or surgical complications. Also, many individuals have monocular vision—good vision in one eye, but little or no vision in the other.

Many individuals with vision impairments can successfully and safely perform their jobs, with or without reasonable accommodation. Under the ADA, these individuals should not be denied employment opportunities for which they are qualified based on stereotypes or incorrect assumptions that they may cause safety hazards, increase employment costs (whether related to the provision of reasonable accommodation or for other reasons), or have difficulty performing certain job duties.

OBTAINING, USING, AND DISCLOSING MEDICAL INFORMATION

The ADA limits an employer's ability to ask questions related to disabilities (including visual disabilities) and to conduct medical examinations. Different rules apply for these inquiries and exams at three distinct stages:

- pre-offer
- post-offer
- during employment

KEEPING MEDICAL INFORMATION CONFIDENTIAL

With limited exceptions, an employer must keep confidential any medical information it learns about an applicant or employee. Under the following circumstances, however, an employer may disclose that an employee has a vision impairment:

- to supervisors and managers, if necessary to provide a reasonable accommodation or meet an employee's work restrictions
- to first aid and safety personnel, if an employee may need emergency treatment or require some other assistance at work
- to individuals investigating compliance with the ADA and similar state and local laws
- when needed for workers' compensation or insurance purposes (e.g., to process a claim)

ACCOMMODATING APPLICANTS AND EMPLOYEES

The ADA requires employers to provide reasonable accommodations in three aspects of employment:

1. Ensuring equal opportunity in the application process.
2. Enabling a qualified individual with a disability to perform the essential functions of their job.
3. Making it possible for an employee with a disability to enjoy equal terms, conditions, benefits, and privileges of employment.

Accommodations vary depending on the needs of the individual with a disability and the situation in which accommodation is needed. Not all applicants or employees with a visual disability will need an accommodation to perform their essential functions or will require the same accommodations to perform the same functions.

CONCERNS ABOUT SAFETY

Regarding safety concerns, an employer should be careful not to act based on myths, fears, or stereotypes about vision impairments. Instead, the employer should evaluate an individual on their skills, knowledge, and experience, and, if any, their disability-related limitations. If the employer has a reasonable belief based on objective evidence that an individual's visual disability may pose safety issues, then it should follow the ADA's "direct threat" analysis, which involves both assessing potential risk and discerning the possibility that reasonable accommodations might reduce or eliminate any such risk.

However, if an employer imposes a vision-related requirement that is necessary to comply with a federal safety law or regulation, the "conflict with other federal laws" defense will apply, and the employer's safety-based qualification standard will be a permissible business necessity under the ADA.

HARASSMENT

The ADA prohibits harassment or offensive conduct based on disability just as other federal laws prohibit harassment based on:

- race
- sex
- color
- national origin
- religion
- age (40 and over)
- genetic information
- pregnancy, childbirth, or related medical conditions

Offensive conduct may include, but is not limited to:

- offensive jokes
- slurs
- epithets or name-calling
- physical assaults or threats
- intimidation
- ridicule or mockery
- insults or put-downs
- offensive music or other sounds
- interference with work performance

Although the law does not prohibit simple teasing, offhand comments, or isolated incidents that are not very serious, harassment is illegal when it is so frequent or severe that it creates a hostile or offensive work environment or when it results in an adverse employment decision (such as the victim being fired or demoted).

RETALIATION AND INTERFERENCE

The ADA prohibits an employer's retaliation against someone who opposes discriminatory employment practices, files a charge of employment discrimination, or testifies or participates in any way in an investigation, proceeding, or litigation related to a charge of employment discrimination. It is also unlawful for an employer to retaliate against someone for requesting a reasonable accommodation or to interfere with the exercise of ADA rights.

The Americans with Disabilities Act (ADA) provides critical protections and guidelines to ensure that individuals with visual disabilities receive fair and equal treatment in the workplace. Employers must understand and comply with these regulations to create an inclusive work environment, addressing the needs and rights of employees with visual disabilities effectively.[1]

Section 28.2 | Employment Protections under the Americans with Disabilities Act and Rehabilitation Act

AMERICANS WITH DISABILITIES ACT

The Americans with Disabilities Act (ADA) prohibits discrimination based on disability in employment, state and local government, public accommodations, commercial facilities, transportation, and telecommunications. It also applies to the United States Congress.

To be protected by the ADA, one must have a disability or have a relationship or association with an individual with a disability.

[1] "Visual Disabilities in the Workplace and the Americans with Disabilities Act," U.S. Equal Employment Opportunity Commission (EEOC), July 26, 2023. Available online. URL: www.eeoc.gov/laws/guidance/visual-disabilities-workplace-and-americans-disabilities-act. Accessed August 7, 2024.

The ADA defines an individual with a disability as a person who has a physical or mental impairment that substantially limits one or more major life activities, a person who has a history or record of such an impairment, or a person who is perceived by others as having such an impairment. The ADA does not specifically name all the impairments that are covered.

ADA Title I: Employment

Title I requires employers with 15 or more employees to provide qualified individuals with disabilities an equal opportunity to benefit from the full range of employment-related opportunities available to others. For example, it prohibits discrimination in:

- recruitment
- hiring
- promotions
- training
- pay
- social activities
- other privileges of employment

It restricts questions that can be asked about an applicant's disability before a job offer is made, and it requires that employers make reasonable accommodations to the known physical or mental limitations of otherwise qualified individuals with disabilities, unless it results in undue hardship. Religious entities with 15 or more employees are covered under Title I.

Title I complaints must be filed with the U.S. Equal Employment Opportunity Commission (EEOC) within 180 days of the date of discrimination, or 300 days if the charge is filed with a designated state or local fair employment practice agency. Individuals may file a lawsuit in federal court only after they receive a "right-to-sue" letter from the EEOC.

Charges of employment discrimination based on disability may be filed at any U.S. Equal Employment Opportunity Commission field office. Field offices are located in 50 cities throughout the United States and are listed in most telephone directories under "U.S. Government."

REHABILITATION ACT

The Rehabilitation Act prohibits employment discrimination based on disability in programs conducted by federal agencies, programs receiving federal financial assistance, federal employment, and the employment practices of federal contractors. The standards for determining employment discrimination under the Rehabilitation Act are the same as those used in Title I of the Americans with Disabilities Act.

Section 501

Section 501 requires affirmative action and nondiscrimination in employment by federal agencies of the executive branch. Employees should contact their agency's Equal Employment Opportunity Office to obtain more information or to file a complaint.

Section 503

Section 503 requires affirmative action and prohibits employment discrimination by federal government contractors and subcontractors with contracts of more than $10,000.

Section 504

Section 504 states that "no qualified individual with a disability in the United States shall be excluded from, denied the benefits of, or be subjected to discrimination under" any program or activity that either receives federal financial assistance or is conducted by any executive agency or the United States Postal Service.

Each federal agency has its own set of Section 504 regulations that apply to its own programs. Agencies that provide federal financial assistance also have Section 504 regulations covering entities that receive federal aid. Requirements common to these regulations include reasonable accommodation for employees with disabilities, program accessibility, effective communication with people who have hearing or vision disabilities, and accessible new construction and alterations. Each agency is responsible for enforcing its own regulations. Section 504 may also be enforced through private lawsuits. It is not necessary to file a complaint with a federal agency or to receive a "right-to-sue" letter before going to court.

Section 508

Section 508 establishes requirements for electronic and information technology developed, maintained, procured, or used by the federal government. Section 508 requires federal electronic and information technology to be accessible to people with disabilities, including employees and members of the public.

An accessible information technology system is one that can be operated in a variety of ways and does not rely on a single sense or ability of the user. For example, a system that provides output only in visual format may not be accessible to people with visual impairments, and a system that provides output only in audio format may not be accessible to people who are deaf or hard of hearing. Some individuals with disabilities may need accessibility-related software or peripheral devices to use systems that comply with Section 508.

Both the ADA and the Rehabilitation Act provide critical protections against discrimination for individuals with disabilities in the workplace. These laws ensure that qualified individuals with disabilities have equal access to employment opportunities and that workplaces are accessible and accommodating to their needs.[1]

[1] ADA.gov, "Guide to Disability Rights Laws," U.S. Department of Justice (DOJ), February 28, 2020. Available online. URL: www.ada.gov/resources/disability-rights-guide. Accessed August 7, 2024.

Chapter 29 | **Access and Rights to Special Education**

Chapter Contents

Section 29.1 | The Individuals with Disabilities Education Act (IDEA)

OVERVIEW OF INDIVIDUALS WITH DISABILITIES EDUCATION ACT

The Individuals with Disabilities Education Act (IDEA) is a law that ensures a free appropriate public education is available to eligible children with disabilities throughout the nation. It provides special education and related services to those children.

The IDEA governs how states and public agencies provide early intervention, special education, and related services to more than 8 million eligible infants, toddlers, children, and youth with disabilities (as of the school year 2022–2023).

EARLY INTERVENTION AND SPECIAL EDUCATION

Infants and toddlers—birth through age two—with disabilities and their families receive early intervention services under IDEA Part C. Children and youth aged 3 through 21 receive special education and related services under IDEA Part B.

PROGRAMS AUTHORIZED BY THE INDIVIDUALS WITH DISABILITIES EDUCATION ACT

The IDEA authorizes several key programs:

Office of Special Education Programs Formula Grant Programs

Office of Special Education Programs (OSEP) administers three formula grant programs authorized by the IDEA. These formula grants are awarded to states annually to support early intervention services for infants and toddlers with disabilities and their families, preschool children aged 3 through 5, and special education for children and youth with disabilities.

Part B Formula Grants

- Assist states in providing a free appropriate public education in the least restrictive environment for children with disabilities, aged 3 through 21.

- Grants to States Program
    - Authorized by Part B, Section 611 for children aged 3 through 21.
- Preschool Grants Program
    - Authorized by Part B, Section 619 for children aged 3 through 5.

Part C Formula Grants

- Support early intervention services for infants and toddlers.
- Grants for Infants and Families Program
    - Authorized by Part C for infants and toddlers, birth through age 2, and their families.

Discretionary Grants

The U.S. Department of Education awards these grants through a competitive process. The OSEP conducts application reviews through a formal peer review process using a standing panel. Reviewers score applications based on legislative and regulatory requirements and published selection criteria established for the grant programs and projects.

LEGISLATIVE BACKGROUND

Congress reauthorized the IDEA in 2004 and most recently amended it through Public Law 114-95, the Every Student Succeeds Act, in December 2015. In the law, Congress states:

Disability is a natural part of the human experience and in no way diminishes the right of individuals to participate in or contribute to society. Improving educational results for children with disabilities is an essential element of our national policy of ensuring equality of opportunity, full participation, independent living, and economic self-sufficiency for individuals with disabilities.

PURPOSE OF THE INDIVIDUALS WITH DISABILITIES EDUCATION ACT

The stated purpose of the IDEA is:

- to ensure that all children with disabilities have available to them a free appropriate public education that emphasizes

special education and related services designed to meet their unique needs and prepare them for:
    - further education
    - employment
    - independent living
- to ensure that the rights of children with disabilities and parents of such children are protected
- to assist states, localities, educational service agencies, and federal agencies in providing for the education of all children with disabilities
- to assist states in the implementation of a statewide, comprehensive, coordinated, multidisciplinary, interagency system of early intervention services for infants and toddlers with disabilities and their families
- to ensure that educators and parents have the necessary tools to improve educational results for children with disabilities by supporting:
    - system improvement activities
    - coordinated research and personnel preparation
    - coordinated technical assistance, dissemination, and support
    - technology development and media services
- to assess and ensure the effectiveness of efforts to educate children with disabilities

The IDEA plays a crucial role in supporting the education and development of children with disabilities. Providing early intervention, special education, and related services ensures these children receive the support they need to achieve their full potential and lead independent, fulfilling lives.[1]

[1] "About IDEA," U.S. Department of Education (ED), December 15, 2015. Available online. URL: https://sites.ed.gov/idea/about-idea. Accessed August 7, 2024.

Section 29.2 | Individualized Education Program (IEP)

WHAT IS AN INDIVIDUALIZED EDUCATION PROGRAM?

Each public school child who receives special education and related services must have an Individualized Education Program (IEP). Each IEP must be designed for one student and must be a truly individualized document. The IEP creates an opportunity for teachers, parents, school administrators, related services personnel, and students (when appropriate) to work together to improve educational results for children with disabilities. The IEP is the cornerstone of a quality education for each child with a disability.

PROCESS OF INDIVIDUALIZED EDUCATION PROGRAM

Step 1: Child Is Identified as Possibly Needing Special Education and Related Services

- **Child Find.** The state must identify, locate, and evaluate all children with disabilities in the state who need special education and related services. To do so, states conduct Child Find activities. A child may be identified by Child Find, and parents may be asked if the Child Find system can evaluate their child. Parents can also call the Child Find system and ask that their child be evaluated.
- **Referral or request for evaluation.** A school professional may ask that a child be evaluated to see if he or she has a disability. Parents may also contact the child's teacher or other school professional to ask that their child be evaluated. This request may be verbal or in writing. Parental consent is needed before the child may be evaluated. Evaluation needs to be completed within a reasonable time after the parent gives consent.

Step 2: Child Is Evaluated

The evaluation must assess the child in all areas related to the child's suspected disability. The evaluation results will be used to decide the child's eligibility for special education and related services and to make decisions about an appropriate educational program for the child. If the parents disagree with the evaluation, they can take their child for an Independent Educational Evaluation (IEE) and ask that the school system pay for this IEE.

Step 3: Eligibility Is Decided

A group of qualified professionals and the parents look at the child's evaluation results. Together, they decide if the child is a "child with a disability," as defined by IDEA. Parents may ask for a hearing to challenge the eligibility decision.

Step 4: The Child Is Found Eligible for Services

If the child is found to be a "child with a disability," as defined by IDEA, he or she is eligible for special education and related services. Within 30 calendar days after a child is determined eligible, the IEP team must meet to write an IEP for the child.

Step 5: Individualized Education Program Meeting Is Scheduled

The school system schedules and conducts the IEP meeting. School staff must:

- contact the participants, including the parents
- notify parents early enough to make sure they have an opportunity to attend
- schedule the meeting at a time and place agreeable to parents and the school
- inform the parents of the purpose, time, and location of the meeting
- tell the parents who will be attending
- tell the parents that they may invite people to the meeting who have knowledge or special expertise about the child

Step 6: Individualized Education Program Meeting Is Held, and the Individualized Education Program Is Written

The IEP team gathers to discuss the child's needs and write the student's IEP. Parents and the student (when appropriate) are part of the team. If a different group decides the child's placement, the parents must be part of that group as well.

The parents must give consent before the school system may provide special education and related services to the child for the first time. The child begins to receive services as soon as possible after the meeting.

If the parents do not agree with the IEP and placement, they may discuss their concerns with other members of the IEP team and try to work out an agreement. If they still disagree, parents can ask for mediation, or the school may offer mediation. Parents may file a complaint with the state education agency and may request a due process hearing, at which time mediation must be available.

Step 7: Services Are Provided

The school ensures that the child's IEP is being carried out as it was written. Parents are given a copy of the IEP. Each of the child's teachers and service providers has access to the IEP and knows his or her specific responsibilities for carrying it out. This includes the accommodations, modifications, and supports that must be provided to the child in keeping with the IEP.

Step 8: Progress Is Measured and Reported to Parents

The child's progress toward the annual goals is measured, as stated in the IEP. His or her parents are regularly informed of their child's progress and whether that progress is enough for the child to achieve the goals by the end of the year. These progress reports must be given to parents at least as often as parents are informed of their nondisabled children's progress.

Step 9: Individualized Education Program Is Reviewed

The child's IEP is reviewed by the IEP team at least once a year, or more often if the parents or school ask for a review. If necessary, the IEP is revised. Parents, as team members, must be invited to attend these meetings. Parents can make suggestions for changes, agree or disagree with the IEP goals, and agree or disagree with the placement.

If parents do not agree with the IEP and placement, they may discuss their concerns with other members of the IEP team and try to work out an agreement. There are several options, including additional testing, an independent evaluation, asking for mediation (if available), or a due process hearing. They may also file a complaint with the state education agency.

Step 10: Child Is Reevaluated

The child must be reevaluated at least every three years. This evaluation is often called a "triennial." Its purpose is to determine whether the child continues to be a "child with a disability," as defined by IDEA, and what the child's educational needs are. However, the child must be reevaluated more often if conditions warrant or if the child's parent or teacher asks for a new evaluation.

If the child is blind or visually impaired, the IEP team shall provide for instruction in Braille or the use of Braille, unless it determines after an appropriate evaluation that the child does not need this instruction.[1]

[1] "A Guide to the Individualized Education Program," U.S. Department of Education (ED), August 30, 2019. Available online. URL: www2.ed.gov/parents/needs/speced/iepguide/index.html. Accessed August 7, 2024.

Chapter 30 | **Benefits and Support Services for Vision Impairment**

Chapter Contents

Section 30.1 | Social Security Benefits for People with Visual Impairments

IF YOU ARE BLIND OR HAVE LOW VISION

You Can Get Disability Benefits If You Are Blind

If you are blind, you may be eligible for Social Security Disability Insurance (SSDI) benefits or Supplemental Security Income (SSI) payments. You are considered blind if your vision cannot be corrected to better than 20/200 in your better eye. You are also considered blind if your visual field is 20 degrees or fewer in your better eye for a period that lasts or is expected to last at least 12 months. The duration requirement does not apply for SSI payments.

You Can Get Disability Benefits Even If You Are Not Blind

If your vision does not meet the definition of blindness, you may still be eligible for disability benefits. This is true if your vision problems alone or combined with other health problems prevent you from working. For SSDI benefits, you must also have worked long enough in a job that paid Social Security taxes. For SSI payments based on disability and blindness, prior work is not required, but your income and resources must be under certain dollar limits.

How You Become Eligible for Social Security Disability Insurance Benefits

When you work and pay Social Security taxes, you earn credits that count toward future SSDI benefits.

If you are blind, you can earn credits anytime during your working years. Credits for your work after becoming blind can help you become eligible for benefits if you do not have enough credits when you become blind. If you do not have enough credits to get SSDI benefits based on your earnings, you may be able to get benefits based on the earnings of a parent or spouse.

Disability Freeze

There is a special rule that may help you eventually get higher retirement or disability benefits. You can use this rule if you are blind but are not getting disability benefits now because you are still working. If your earnings are lower because of your blindness, the years when you earned less can be excluded when calculating your Social Security retirement or disability benefit in the future. This rule is called a "disability freeze." Contact Social Security to file for this "freeze."

You Can Get SSI Payments

The SSI program is a needs-based program. Your income and resources must be less than certain dollar limits, which vary from state to state. You do not need to have worked under Social Security to qualify for SSI. Ask your local Social Security office about the income and resource limits in your state and read SSI (Publication No. 05-11000).

YOU CAN WORK WHILE RECEIVING BENEFITS

Work incentives make it easier for people receiving disability benefits to work.

People receiving SSDI benefits can continue to receive them when they work, as long as their earnings do not exceed an amount set by law.

If you are receiving SSDI benefits and are blind, you can earn as much as $2,590 per month in 2024. This is higher than the earnings limit of $1,550 per month, which applies to workers with disabilities who are not blind. The earnings limit usually changes each year. Additionally, if you are blind and self-employed, the time spent working in your business is not evaluated as it is for people who are not blind. This means you can work for your business and still receive disability benefits if your net profit averages $2,590 or less monthly in 2024.

Work Is Figured Differently Beginning at Age 55

If you are 55 or older and blind, work determination rules differ from those for people who are not blind. Beginning at age 55, if your earnings exceed $2,590 a month in 2024, benefits are suspended but not terminated. This applies if the work you are doing requires a lower level of skill and ability than what you did before reaching 55. Disability benefits will be paid for any month your earnings fall below this limit.

Different work incentives apply to people receiving SSI.

SPECIAL SERVICES FOR PEOPLE WHO ARE BLIND OR HAVE LOW VISION

Some services and products are designed specifically for people who are blind or have low vision.

Social Security Notices

You can choose to receive notices from Social Security in one of the following ways:

- standard print notice by first-class mail
- standard print notice by certified mail
- standard print notice by first-class mail and a follow-up telephone call
- Braille notice and a standard print notice by first-class mail
- Microsoft Word file on a data Compact Disc (CD) and a standard print notice by first-class mail
- audio CD and a standard print notice by first-class mail
- large print (18-point size) notice and a standard print notice by first-class mail

Several options are available for choosing how to receive notices from Social Security:

- Visit www.ssa.gov/people/blind and follow the steps provided.
- Call toll-free at 800-772-1213. For those who are deaf or hard of hearing, call the teletypewriter (TTY) number at 800-325-0778.
- Write or visit the local Social Security office.

For questions about a Social Security notice, call toll-free at 800-772-1213 to have the notice read or explained.[1]

---

[1] "If You Are Blind or Have Low Vision—How We Can Help," U.S. Social Security Administration (SSA), 2024. Available online. URL: www.ssa.gov/pubs/EN-05-10052.pdf. Accessed August 7, 2024.

Section 30.2 | Free or Low Cost Eye Care

Eye care can be expensive, but fortunately, there are programs offering free or low-cost eye exams and eyeglasses. Some health insurance plans also provide free vision screenings and assist with the cost of other eye care services.

PROGRAMS THAT OFFER FREE OR LOW-COST EYE CARE

These programs offer free or low-cost eye care, though you must apply and meet certain criteria, such as having a low income or a higher risk of certain eye diseases.

Most of these programs operate nationwide, but your area may also have local organizations and services to assist.

For All Ages

- **Your regular doctor**. They may be able to refer you to affordable eye care services.
- **Your eye doctor**. If you have an eye doctor and need help paying for care or treatment, ask about programs for which you may qualify.
- **Community health centers**. Some centers have an eye clinic offering free or low-cost care. Use this tool to find a community health center near you.
- **Local colleges or universities**. If there is an optometry or ophthalmology program nearby, inquire about low-cost eye care options.
- **Your local pharmacy**. Ask your pharmacist about discounts on medicines or medicine delivery services.
- **Additional resources**:
    - VSP Eyes of Hope (www.vspvision.com/cms/vspglobal-outreach/gift-certificates.html) provides children and adults with no-cost eye care and eyeglasses, targeting those with limited income and no health insurance. To apply, you will need assistance from a school nurse or a community partner organization.

- Lions Clubs International (www.lionsclubs.org/en/start-our-approach/club-locator) helps cover eye care costs through its local clubs, some of which may also provide eyeglasses.
- New Eyes (https://new-eyes.org/application) provides prescription eyeglasses to children and adults who cannot afford them. A social worker or someone at a community health center may help you apply.
- Mission Cataract USA (https://missioncataractusa.org/doctors) offers free cataract surgery to people of all ages who cannot afford it.
- Operation Sight (https://ascrs.org/foundation/operation-sight/patient-inquiry) assists people with low incomes in obtaining cataract surgery.
- The American Glaucoma Society (www.americanglaucomasociety.net/patients/ags-cares) supports individuals with low incomes or no insurance in obtaining glaucoma surgery through its AGS Cares program.
- The National Federation of the Blind (https://nfb.org/programs-services/free-white-cane-program) provides free white canes for personal use.
- Prevent Blindness (https://preventblindness.org/vision-care-financial-assistance-information) has a comprehensive list of organizations and services that provide financial assistance for vision care.

For Older Adults

- EyeCare America (https://secure.aao.org/Forms/ECAReferral) offers free comprehensive eye exams and up to one year of care to people aged 65 and older and to those at higher risk of glaucoma.

For Children

- All Children See (www.childrenseyefoundation.org/webdev/what-we-do/all-children-see/all-children-see-patients) connects you with eye doctors that can provide a comprehensive eye exam. Children qualify for the program if they had a vision

screening that identified an eye problem or if they show signs of vision issues. Note this program is only available in some states.
- InfantSEE (www.infantsee.org/find-a-doctor?sso=y) offers free eye assessments for babies aged 6 to 12 months. An eye doctor conducts these assessments and may identify problems that a regular vision check would not.

HEALTH INSURANCE AND EYE CARE

Under the Affordable Care Act, many health insurance plans are required to cover the full cost of vision screenings for children and teens (up to age 19). Health insurance plans may also help cover the cost of eye care for eye diseases such as cataracts, diabetic eye disease, and glaucoma.

Medicaid, Children's Health Insurance Program, and Medicare

- Medicaid and Children's Health Insurance Program (CHIP; www.insurekidsnow.gov/coverage/index.html) offer free or low-cost health insurance for children from families with low incomes. These programs cover the cost of vision care for children, though each state has different eligibility rules.
- Medicare is a government health insurance program for people aged 65 and older and some people younger than 65 with disabilities. It does not cover routine eye exams or eyeglasses for most people, but it does help cover some eye care costs for those with:
  - diabetes (www.medicare.gov/coverage/eye-exams-for-diabetes)
  - age-related macular degeneration (AMD; www.medicare.gov/coverage/macular-degeneration-tests-treatment)
  - a high risk of glaucoma (www.medicare.gov/coverage/glaucoma-tests)
  - cataracts (www.medicare.gov/coverage/eyeglasses-contact-lenses)

If you need help understanding your Medicare benefits or coverage, contact your State Health Insurance Assistance Program (SHIP; www.shiphelp.org/about-medicare/regional-ship-location).

Veterans Affairs Health Care

If you are a Veteran or service member qualified for health benefits through the U.S. Department of Veterans Affairs (VA; www.va.gov/health-care/about-va-health-benefits/vision-care), the VA will cover routine eye exams and preventive vision testing (e.g., for glaucoma). You may also be able to get eyeglasses and other necessary vision care covered through the VA.

Other Health Insurance Plans

If you enroll in a health insurance plan through the National Health Insurance Marketplace or a state Marketplace or Exchange, your plan covers free vision screenings for children and teens. Many private health insurance plans—such as those offered by your employer—also provide free vision screenings for children.

Before visiting the eye doctor, it is a good idea to confirm whether a comprehensive eye exam is covered under your health insurance plan.[1]

Section 30.3 | Supplemental Security Income (SSI)

WHAT IS SUPPLEMENTAL SECURITY INCOME?

Supplemental Security Income (SSI) provides monthly payments to adults and children who have income and resources below specific financial thresholds and who meet one of the following criteria:

- They are 65 years of age or older.
- They are blind.
- They have a medical condition that prevents them from working, which is expected to last at least one year or result in death.

[1] "Get Free or Low-Cost Eye Care," National Eye Institute (NEI), April 25, 2022. Available online. URL: www.nei.nih.gov/learn-about-eye-health/healthy-vision/get-free-or-low-cost-eye-care. Accessed August 7, 2024.

If you apply for SSI, you should also review *What You Need To Know When You Get Supplemental Security Income* (Publication No. 05-11011).

Note: *Children with a qualifying disability or blindness and whose parents have low incomes or limited resources may also be eligible for SSI. The basic SSI payment is consistent nationwide, although many states provide additional funds. You can contact SSI to find out the amounts in your state.*

HOW TO APPLY FOR SUPPLEMENTAL SECURITY INCOME

You can begin the application process for SSI and complete a significant portion of your application by visiting this web page: www.ssa.gov/ssi.

If you are an adult with a disability intending to file for both SSI and Social Security Disability Insurance (SSDI), you can apply online for both benefits simultaneously if you meet the following requirements:

- You are between the ages of 18 and 65.
- You have never been married.
- You are a U.S. citizen residing in 1 of the 50 states, the District of Columbia, or the Northern Mariana Islands.
- You have not previously applied for or received SSI.

To apply for both SSI and SSDI online, visit this web page: www.ssa.gov/disability.

Another way to start your application is to use an online tool at this web page: www.ssa.gov/benefits/ssi/start.html. The process takes approximately 5–10 minutes, and no documentation is required initially. SSI will need information about you and, if applicable, about the person you are assisting.

Information Needed from Applicants

- name
- date of birth
- Social Security number

- mailing address
- phone number
- email address (optional)

If you are assisting another person, SSI will also need your name, phone number, and email address (optional).

After completing the online process, a Social Security representative will schedule an appointment to help you apply for benefits. SSI will send an appointment date and time by mail (and by email, if provided) within 7–14 business days.

If you cannot apply online, you can call SSI toll-free at 800-772-1213 to set up an appointment with your local Social Security office. If you are deaf or hard of hearing, you can call SSI at teletypewriter (TTY) number, 800-325-0778.

Parents or guardians can usually apply on behalf of children under age 18 who are blind or have a disability. In some cases, other third parties may apply on behalf of children.

Items to Bring When Applying

- Social Security card or a record of your Social Security number
- birth certificate or other proof of age
- information about your residence, such as a mortgage or lease along with your landlord's name
- payroll slips, bank books, insurance policies, burial fund records, and other information about your income and assets
- names, addresses, and phone numbers of medical sources, if applying due to a disability or blindness
- proof of U.S. citizenship or eligible noncitizen status
- your checkbook or other papers that show your bank, credit union, or savings and loan account number

If approved for SSI, you must receive your payments electronically. Payments can be made via direct deposit, the Direct Express® card program, or an Electronic Transfer Account. For more information, visit this website: www.GoDirect.org.

A Note for People Who Are Blind or Have a Qualifying Disability

If you are blind or have a qualifying disability and are employed, special rules may allow you to continue receiving SSI payments while you work. As your earnings increase, your SSI payments may be reduced or stopped, but you may be able to maintain your Medicaid coverage.

You may also be able to set aside money for work-related goals or education without reducing your SSI payment. Individuals who are blind or have a qualifying disability and are applying for SSI may receive special services to assist with employment, such as counseling, job training, and job placement support.

For more information, consult *Working While Disabled—How We Can Help* (Publication No. 05-10095).

RIGHT TO APPEAL

If you disagree with a decision made on your claim, you have the right to appeal. The necessary steps are detailed in *Your Right To Question The Decision Made On Your Claim* (Publication No. 05-10058).

You may manage your own SSI case or appeal with free assistance from SSI. You also have the right to have someone represent you. There are specific rules about who can represent you and what your representative can do. SSI will interact with your representative as SSI would with you directly. For more information on appointing a representative, refer to *Your Right To Representation* (Publication No. 05-10075) or visit this web page: www.ssa.gov/representation.

Additional Assistance

If you receive SSI, you may also qualify for additional support from your state or county, such as Medicaid, food assistance, or other social services. Contact your local social services department or public welfare office for information about services available in your community.[1]

---

[1] "Supplemental Security Income (SSI)," U.S. Social Security Administration (SSA), May 15, 2023. Available online. URL: www.ssa.gov/pubs/EN-05-11000.pdf. Accessed August 7, 2024.

Section 30.4 | Supplemental Nutrition Assistance Program (SNAP)

WHAT IS SUPPLEMENTAL NUTRITION ASSISTANCE PROGRAM?

The Supplemental Nutrition Assistance Program (SNAP), formerly known as "food stamps," assists low-income individuals and families in purchasing nutritious food. While SNAP is a federal program, it is administered by state agencies through local offices. If you meet certain income and resource criteria, you may be eligible for SNAP benefits.

CAN YOU GET SUPPLEMENTAL NUTRITION ASSISTANCE PROGRAM?

To qualify for SNAP benefits, your household must meet specific conditions and requirements. A household includes everyone who lives with you and shares both the purchase and preparation of meals.

If you are homeless, you are still eligible for SNAP benefits even without a permanent address, a stable place to stay, or a facility to cook meals. You are considered homeless if you:

- do not have a fixed, regular nighttime residence
- primarily reside overnight in temporary accommodation, including a supervised shelter, halfway house, the residence of another person, or a nontraditional sleeping area such as a hallway, bus station, or lobby

HOW CAN YOU APPLY FOR SUPPLEMENTAL NUTRITION ASSISTANCE PROGRAM?

Applications for SNAP benefits are available at any Social Security office. If you and everyone in your household are applying for or already receiving Supplemental Security Income (SSI) payments, any Social Security office can assist you in filling out the SNAP application and forwarding it to the SNAP office on your behalf.

All other applicants, including those only receiving Social Security benefits, must submit their applications directly to their local

SNAP office. To locate your nearest SNAP office or to apply online, visit this web page: www.fns.usda.gov/snap/state-directory. Alternatively, you can contact the SNAP information line toll-free at 800-221-5689.

After submitting your application, you must complete an interview, which, in most cases, can be conducted by telephone. Along with the application and interview, you must provide verification of certain information. Documents to verify information on your SNAP application may include:

- identification such as a driver's license, state ID card, birth certificate, work or school ID card, health insurance card, voter registration card, or proof of alien status
- proof of income for each household member, including pay stubs, employer statements, current benefit verification letters from Social Security, veteran's benefits, unemployment insurance, and documentation of child support or alimony
- proof of dependent care expenses
- rent receipts or mortgage payment records
- utility cost records
- medical bills for household members aged 60 or older, and for those receiving disability benefits such as Social Security Disability or SSI

The SNAP office processing your application will determine if your household qualifies for benefits. You should receive a decision within 30 days. Households eligible for expedited service may receive benefits within seven days. If you do not receive a response within 30 days after applying, contact or visit the SNAP office.

HOW MUCH CAN YOU GET?

The amount of SNAP benefits your household receives depends on its size, monthly income, and expenses such as mortgage or rent, utilities, and childcare or elder care that enable employment.

For more information or to apply online, visit this web page: www.fns.usda.gov/snap/state-directory. You can also contact the SNAP information line toll-free at 800-221-5689. To learn about other nutrition assistance programs that may be available, consult

Nutrition Assistance Programs (Publication No. 05-10100) or visit this website: www.fns.usda.gov.[1]

Section 30.5 | Disability Benefits for Children

WHAT IS SUPPLEMENTAL SECURITY INCOME?

Supplemental Security Income (SSI) provides monthly payments to individuals with limited income and resources who are 65 or older, blind, or disabled. Children under the age of 18 may be eligible if they have a medical condition or a combination of conditions that meet Social Security's definition of disability, and their income and resources fall within the eligibility limits. The amount of the SSI payment varies from state to state because some states supplement the federal SSI payment. Local Social Security offices can provide more information about state-specific total SSI payments.

SUPPLEMENTAL SECURITY INCOME RULES ABOUT INCOME AND RESOURCES

Eligibility for SSI considers the income and resources of both the child and the family members if they reside in the child's household. This applies whether the child lives at home or is away at school but returns home occasionally and remains under parental control. If the income and resources exceed the allowable amount, the application for SSI payments will be denied. Children in a medical facility where health insurance pays for their care receive a limited monthly SSI payment of $30.

SUPPLEMENTAL SECURITY INCOME RULES ABOUT DISABILITY

To be medically eligible for SSI, a child must meet all the following disability requirements:

- If not blind, the child must not work or earn more than $1,550 a month in 2024. If blind, the earning

[1] "Supplemental Nutrition Assistance Program (SNAP) Facts," U.S. Social Security Administration (SSA), December 1, 2022. Available online. URL: www.ssa.gov/pubs/EN-05-10101.pdf. Accessed August 7, 2024.

limit is $2,590. These amounts typically adjust annually.
- The child must have a medical condition or a combination of conditions that result in "marked and severe functional limitations," meaning the conditions seriously limit the child's activities.
- The condition(s) must have been or be expected to be disabling for at least 12 months, or expected to result in death.

PROVIDING INFORMATION ABOUT YOUR CHILD'S CONDITION

When applying for SSI on behalf of a child, detailed information about the child's medical condition and its effect on daily activities is required. Doctors, teachers, therapists, and other professionals who have information about the child's condition must also be given permission to send the information. Submitting any available medical or school records can help expedite the decision-making process.

WHAT HAPPENS NEXT?

After submission, the information is forwarded to the Disability Determination Services (DDS) in the respective state. DDS professionals will review the child's medical and school records and other necessary information to determine if the child meets the disability criteria. If the information provided is insufficient, DDS may require a medical examination or test for the child, which will be funded. The decision process by the state agency can take between six and eight months.

SUPPLEMENTAL SECURITY INCOME DISABILITY REVIEWS

Once a child starts receiving SSI, periodic reviews of their medical condition are legally required to ensure it still meets the disability criteria:

- Reviews occur at least every three years for children under 18 whose conditions are expected to improve or where improvement is possible.

- For infants receiving SSI due to low birth weight, a review happens by their first birthday unless their condition is not expected to improve by that time, in which case the review may be postponed.

During these reviews, evidence that the child's disability continues to severely limit daily activities and that they are receiving medically necessary treatment must be presented.

WHAT HAPPENS WHEN A CHILD TURNS 18?

In the SSI program, an individual is considered an adult at 18, and different medical and nonmedical rules are applied to determine eligibility for SSI disability payments. For instance, the income and resources of family members, except for a spouse, are no longer counted. Adult disability rules are applied to determine the disability status.

- If a child already receives SSI payments, their medical condition is reviewed using adult disability rules within the year following their 18th birthday to decide if they remain eligible for SSI.
- If a child was not eligible for SSI before their 18th birthday due to family income or resources, they might become eligible at 18.

DETERMINING SOCIAL SECURITY DISABILITY INSURANCE ELIGIBILITY FOR ADULTS OVER 18

For those aged 18 or older, disability is assessed similarly to any adult. Applications are forwarded to the state's DDS, which determines the disability.[1]

[1] "Benefits for Children with Disabilities," U.S. Social Security Administration (SSA), January 2, 2024. Available online. URL: www.ssa.gov/pubs/EN-05-10026.pdf. Accessed August 7, 2024.

Part 5 | **Additional Resources**

Chapter 31 | Directory of Organizations Providing Support for People with Visual Impairments

Americans with Disabilities Act (ADA)
Toll-Free: 800-514-0301
Toll-Free TTY: 800-514-0383
Website: www.ada.gov

Centers for Disease Control and Prevention (CDC)
1600 Clifton Rd., N.E.
Atlanta, GA 30329-4027
Toll-Free: 800-CDC-INFO (800-232-4636)
Phone: 770-488-1725
Toll-Free TTY: 888-232-6348
Website: www.cdc.gov
Email: hrcs@cdc.gov

Genetic and Rare Diseases Information Center (GARD)
P.O. Box 8126
Gaithersburg, MD 20898-8126
Toll-Free: 888-205-2311
Toll-Free TTY: 888-205-3223
Fax: 301-251-4911
Website: https://rarediseases.info.nih.gov

Resources in this chapter were compiled from several sources deemed reliable; all contact information was verified and updated in August 2024.

MedlinePlus
8600 Rockville Pike
Bethesda, MD 20894
Website: https://medlineplus.gov

National Cancer Institute (NCI)
9609 Medical Center Dr.
Bethesda, MD 20892-9760
Toll-Free: 800-4-CANCER (800-422-6237)
Website: www.cancer.gov
Email: NCIinfo@nih.gov

National Eye Institute (NEI)
31 Center Dr., MSC 2510
Bethesda, MD 20892-2510
Phone: 301-496-5248
Website: www.nei.nih.gov
Email: 2020@nei.nih.gov

National Institute of Biomedical Imaging and Bioengineering (NIBIB)
9000 Rockville Pike, Bldg. 31
Rm. 1C14
Bethesda, MD 20892
Phone: 301-496-8859
Website: www.nibib.nih.gov
Email: info@nibib.nih.gov

National Institute on Aging (NIA)
P.O. Box 8057
Gaithersburg, MD 20898
Toll-Free: 800-222-2225
Website: www.nia.nih.gov
Email: niaic@nia.nih.gov

National Institutes of Health (NIH)
9000 Rockville Pike
Bethesda, MD 20892
Phone: 301-496-4000
TTY: 301-402-9612
Website: www.nih.gov

U.S. Department of Transportation (DOT)

1200 New Jersey Ave., S.E.
Washington, DC 20590
Toll-Free: 855-368-4200
Phone: 202-366-4000
Website: www.transportation.gov

U.S. Department of Veterans Affairs (VA)

Toll-Free: 844-698-2311
Website: www.va.gov

U.S. Social Security Administration (SSA)

P.O. Box 17769
Baltimore, MD 21235-7769
Toll-Free: 800-772-1213
Toll-Free TTY: 800-325-0778
Website: www.ssa.gov

INDEX

INDEX

Page numbers followed by "n" refer to citation information; by "t" indicate tables; and by "f" indicate figures.

D

E

F

O

P

Q

R

S